D1142462

DIRECTORY OF

Complementary Therapy Services

in UK Cancer Care

PUBLIC AND VOLUNTARY SECTORS

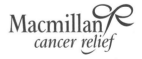

Our vision

Imagine a time when every person in the land has equal and ready access to the best information, treatment and care for cancer and unnecessary levels of fear are set aside

At Macmillan Cancer Relief we dedicate ourselves to working with others to turn this vision into everyone's reality.

Published by Macmillan Cancer Relief in association with Cambridge Publishers.
© Macmillan Cancer Relief 2002. Designed by Belinda Magee.

Registered Office 89 Albert Embankment, London SE1 7UQ
Tel: 020 7840 7840 Fax: 020 7840 7841 **Macmillan CancerLine 0808 808 2020**
www.macmillan.org.uk   Registered Charity Number 261017

ISBN 0 9536785 2 0

One of the pleasures of my association with Macmillan Cancer Relief has been to see how innovative ideas can evolve into practical action to improve the quality of life for cancer patients and their carers.

It hardly needs saying that cancer can have a devastating impact on individuals, their families and friends. Having easy access to good support services, as well as effective medical treatment, can make all the difference to the way people cope with the disease. It can help them think more positively about their future too. Complementary therapies can provide emotional and psychological support to patients, not just relieve their physical symptoms. Indeed, friends of mine have repeatedly told me how much better they have felt as a result of receiving such therapies alongside orthodox cancer care.

I am delighted, therefore, that Macmillan has recognised the needs expressed by many patients and healthcare professionals for guidance about services available in their areas - and acted to help meet them. This first directory of complementary therapy services in UK cancer care demonstrates Macmillan's commitment to developing practical solutions to common problems. I hope that it serves to increase and inform choices open to people with cancer, and encourage wider access to treatments that they find comforting and beneficial.

Increasingly, people want compassionate healthcare for themselves and their families; treatments that engage the mind, or calm troubled spirits as well as heal the body. Long may Macmillan continue to promote and illuminate this compassionate approach in our health services

66 The majority of cancer patients at some stage of their illness will explore the use of complementary therapies. This term covers an ever burgeoning range of treatments, few of which have been properly evaluated and most of which are unregulated. There is an urgent need for reliable information about this area with some sensible advice on how to use it. This directory from Macmillan provides a unique contribution to this process and I am sure will be helpful not just to patients and families but to their professional carers also. 99

Professor Geoff Hanks,
Professor of Palliative Medicine,
Bristol Haematology and Oncology Centre

66 This directory guides the patient to the rightful place of complementary medicine. Provided that the complementary specialist concentrates on making the patient feel better and spiritually at ease, then its position is secure into the new millennium. 99

Professor Michael Baum,
Emeritus Professor of Surgery,
University College London

66 This is what every professional needs to hand when they see patients. 99

Dr Jane Maher, Chief Medical Officer, Macmillan Cancer Relief

66 Complementary therapies have the potential to greatly enhance the patient's experience of their cancer journey. I am very pleased that Macmillan is providing this resource to health professionals around the country. 99

Dr Greg Tanner, Macmillan GP Adviser
and National Clinical Lead for Primary Care
for the Cancer Services Collaborative

66 If we are truly caring for the whole person, we cannot ignore the enormous benefits that complementary therapies can bring to our patients and, directly or indirectly, their families and carers. 99

Dr Cath Dyer, Macmillan Lead GP

66 I am delighted that this directory has been published by Macmillan Cancer Relief. The benefits of complementary therapies are now very well established, enhancing quality of life and sense of wellbeing both during and following treatments for cancer. This will be an excellent resource across the whole of the country. 99

Judith Spencer-Knott,
Macmillan Breast Care Specialist Nurse

Foreword

I am delighted to add my support to this ground-breaking piece of work. Never before has quite so much local information about complementary therapies been brought together in one place.

This directory marks the culmination of a period of intense activity from not only staff and postholders within Macmillan Cancer Relief but our friends and colleagues too. Our earlier work made clear that all people, but particularly those living with cancer are increasingly finding benefit from a range of complementary therapies. The difficulty was discovering where such support might be found. This directory is that first step and, to quote Lao-tzu 'a journey of 1000 miles starts with just one step'. We look forward to this volume being used by individuals, professionals, information centres and help lines.

Over time and with your help we can ensure that comprehensive information is available that will allow individuals to make choices and to access the therapies that may really make a difference to living with cancer. I add my congratulations to all those many people involved with this major piece of work and my support to all those who will use it into the future.

Dame Gill Oliver

Director of Service Development

Macmillan Cancer Relief

April 2002

Contents

Introduction

Macmillan Cancer Relief is a UK charity which helps to provide the expert care and practical and emotional support that makes a real difference for people living with cancer.

A vital part of this role is to signpost patients to useful sources of information, and to help provide healthcare professionals with materials to support and inform the guidance they give to their patients. Listening to people with cancer, and service providers, keeps us in touch with changing needs and circumstances.

In 1999, Macmillan Cancer Relief commissioned a study, *Complementary Therapies in Cancer Care*[1], to find out what role these treatments were playing in the care of patients in the UK – and why. The report found complementary therapies were enthusiastically received by patients, for the psychological benefits they offered and for their potential to improve symptom management.

In addition, surveys of Macmillan nurses and doctors showed the overwhelming majority were asked about complementary therapies by their patients and most tried to respond with information and/or advice. However, one of the unmet needs identified in this survey was for reliable information on the availability and range of complementary therapy services in their local areas. There appeared to be no readily accessible source of this knowledge for them or for practitioners or patients. Macmillan was keen to find a way of plugging this knowledge gap with a single, easy-to-use publication. This directory is the result.

It aims to provide up-to-date information about complementary therapies available to cancer patients and their carers in the UK – both in the public and voluntary health sectors. Although we appreciate that this first directory is not fully comprehensive – and the information inevitably may change – we hope that it will serve as a useful starting point for people who want to find out which therapies are available locally.

---

1. *Complementary Therapies in Cancer Care – Abridged report of a study produced for Macmillan Cancer Relief*. Kohn M, 1999, Macmillan Cancer Relief

Complementary therapies – definition and evidence

Complementary therapies have been described and defined in several ways in the research literature. For the purposes of this directory, we define them as therapies that can work alongside, and in combination with, orthodox medical treatment. A range of different methods may be applied in this group of therapies, including complete healing systems, such as homeopathy and acupuncture; techniques like massage and reflexology; and self-care approaches – such as meditation and diet. A full list of the therapies and the rationale for their inclusion can be found in Appendix 1 and Appendix 3 respectively.

Scientific and anecdotal evidence for using complementary therapies

Complementary therapies have become a significant feature of healthcare practice in the UK over the past decade. Many hospital oncology units, and hospices, offer at least one complementary therapy, usually as an adjunct to conventional care. Although the scientific evidence base for complementary therapies is still small, this does not mean that they are ineffective. Rather it reflects the fact that only limited resources have been committed to research, and that many clinical trials have been of poor methodological quality. We do not evaluate the efficacy of individual therapies in this directory. Such assessments are documented in other texts, and we recommend that readers consult at least some of these to satisfy themselves that a therapy is worth pursuing. Details of further reading material are available in Appendix 2.

However, anecdotal evidence suggests that many people find complementary therapies help them cope with the experience of cancer. Patients and their carers frequently report reduced anxiety, less depression, greater relaxation, better sleep, better symptom control (less pain and nausea, for example) and an improved sense of well-being after complementary treatment.

How complementary therapies can help patients during their cancer journey

" It's acupuncture that's helped me to cope with the chemo."

Maggie on the reduction in nausea she experiences since she started having acupuncture before each chemotherapy treatment

" I've learnt to carry on the relaxation at home too. I sleep better and don't get so worked up."

Arthur, who attends a weekly relaxation group

" Massage simply makes me feel better and more able to cope."

Rose, whose husband has cancer

" When I first decided to ask for healing, I had no idea what to expect. When it started, I began to calm down a little; I realised this was my time to receive and that I was beginning to connect with my inner feelings and acknowledge my emotions. After about four sessions I began to feel huge surges of energy and I learned to direct and use this energy myself and to call upon it when I needed it."

Sally, aged 29

" I went in (as) one woman and came out another."

Annie on her sense of well-being following an aromatherapy massage

" I sleep really well, I am so relaxed afterwards."

Roy describing reflexology

" It's my oasis. I can say anything to her – I can have a bad day and it's OK."

Eleanor describing time with a counsellor

Making professional judgements about complementary therapies

How can professionals know who might really benefit from undergoing a complementary therapy? When the evidence for its role in alleviating specific conditions is limited, this may not be an easy professional judgement to make. Aside from promoting general well-being, possible reasons why patients may seek complementary therapies include:

- Physical symptoms caused by the disease such as pain, nausea, fatigue
- Need for support during (conventional) treatment
- Advanced cancer
- Loss of confidence, sense of control
- Depression
- Acute or chronic anxiety or panic attacks
- Poor body image
- Insomnia

What patients should consider before trying a complementary therapy

A patient doesn't necessarily have to be referred by a nurse or doctor to try a complementary therapy. He or she can find their own therapist and make an appointment. However, Macmillan recommends that cancer patients consult the healthcare professional in overall charge of their care, or the doctor or nurse that they see most often. Such discussion can help patients decide which therapy or therapist is most likely to help meet their individual needs.

No reputable complementary therapist would claim to be able to cure cancer. Research is being conducted to find out whether some complementary therapies can actually treat cancer, but this is still very much in its infancy.

On the right is a checklist of practical steps that Macmillan recommends patients take to reassure themselves, before trying out a particular therapy or therapist. These draw on guidance issued by several cancer organisations.

DO ...

- Establish what the therapy is intended to achieve

- Use a therapist who has a recognised qualification, belongs to a professional body and has insurance. Ask if the person is experienced and/or trained in treating cancer patients

- Ask for an informal chat with the therapist, and/or ask for any leaflets or literature supplied by them

- Find out what the fees are (if any) and what these cover

- Talk to family, friends and health professionals about your plans

- Consult any relevant fact sheets/telephone help lines provided by reputable patient support organisations

- Find out what is available on the NHS: in treatment centres you may already be using or through your family doctor at the Medical Centre. Wherever you are, ask about the availability of the full range of complementary therapy services

DON'T ...

- Abandon proven conventional treatments

- Be misled by promises or suggestions of cures or respond to a 'hard sell' that offers simple solutions

- Rely on a single source of information as it may be inaccurate

- Use a therapist who cannot refer you to the relevant research

- Feel pressured to buy expensive books, videos, nutritional supplements or herbal preparations as part of a therapy

- Be afraid to ask for references and credentials

- Accept treatment from someone who makes you feel uncomfortable in any way.

Personal recommendations are worth having, but should be considered only in addition to the above questions, not instead of them.

Ensuring quality of care

National guidelines for the use of complementary therapies in palliative care are currently being developed by the Foundation for Integrated Medicine (FIM) and the National Council for Hospice and Specialist Palliative Care Services. The guidelines are expected to be available from early 2003 and will focus on complementary therapies most commonly used in palliative care. (FIM's contact details are listed in Appendix 2.) The National Institute for Clinical Excellence (NICE) is planning to review complementary therapies in the Supportive and Palliative Care Guidance.

Bringing complementary therapies closer to home

If patients have been using a complementary therapy in a cancer treatment setting, there may be opportunities for them to continue receiving it in their local area. Some services have developed a network of community-based practitioners who may even treat patients in their own homes. Hospices may offer complementary therapies to cancer patients on a day care basis; GP surgeries may provide some therapies and private practitioners may also be locally available. We recommend that patients inquire about the availability of such services in their areas – but remember to check that the practitioner is properly qualified and experienced.

How to use the directory

We have organised the directory to show which complementary therapy services are available in your local area. You can use the maps to see 'at a glance' which towns and cities near you host one or more complementary health centres. The main part of the directory shows the details of all the providers for each county, giving key information about the services and therapies on offer. Each entry includes the referral criteria involved and the steps taken by providers to ensure a quality service.

Alternatively, you can use the two indexes to see either where a particular therapy is available across the country, or to find a particular centre by name.

The various appendices at the back of the directory describe the characteristics of all the therapies, give lists of relevant organisations, books and other useful resources and contain information about how the publication was compiled.

What if you cannot find services listed for your area?

The information in the directory was obtained by questionnaire; if your local area doesn't feature, it does not necessarily mean that there are no complementary therapy services. It may just mean that the providers in that area did not receive or return their questionnaire.

We suggest that you try contacting the regional and national organisations listed in Appendix 2. Alternatively, you could try telephoning your nearest provider and ask whether they know of any services available in your area.

Access to this directory

Later in the year, we plan to make a version of this directory more widely available to patients and their carers via the Macmillan website. The Macmillan CancerLine (0808 808 2020) will also be able to give callers information from the directory.

We appreciate that some providers may not have received our questionnaire or may have been unable to respond within the requested time. We apologise to any services that would like to have been included and which fall within the scope of the directory. We hope to be able to include their entries in any future editions. The more relevant entries we can publish, the more comprehensive and informative the publication will become in future years.

We encourage feedback from users of the directory on any aspect of the material featured and have enclosed a form for your comments. Alternatively, please e-mail us directly at **ctdirectory@macmillan.org.uk.**

Production of this directory has been very much a collaboration between Macmillan Cancer Relief, partner organisations and other interested parties. We greatly appreciate the tremendous support from all those involved with us in this venture.

Dr Michelle Kohn MB BSc MRCP

Project Chair and Complementary Therapies Medical Adviser

Macmillan Cancer Relief
April 2002

Acknowledgements *We are most grateful to all those individuals who spared their valuable time to contribute to this project. Our thanks go to all those at Macmillan, in particular Grainne Kavanagh and Neil Gordon for their tremendous work in production, assisted by Priti Patel and the Services Administration Team; Dame Gill Oliver and Stephen Richards for their support throughout and Juliet Gilchrist of Cancerlink (now part of Macmillan). We are most indebted to all the other members of the steering group who helped shape this initiative; Lucy Bell, Mezzi Franklin, Penny Jones, John Kapp, Rosemary Lucey and Dr David Peters. A special thank you to Jenny Penson for her guidance, Alex Hall for her administrative help, Cambridge Publishers and Judy Jones for their editorial expertise and to Belinda Magee for her creative input.*

Steering Group

Dr Michelle Kohn Project Chair and Complementary Therapies
Medical Adviser, Macmillan Cancer Relief

Grainne Kavanagh Project Manager and Services Administration Manager,
Macmillan Cancer Relief

Neil Gordon Project Information Manager

Lucy Bell Complementary Therapy Team Leader, Cancer Services,
Hammersmith Hospitals NHS Trust

Mezzi Franklin Hospital Macmillan Clinical Nurse Specialist,
North Devon District Hospital

Juliet Gilchrist Group Support Officer, Cancerlink, now part of
Macmillan Cancer Relief

Penny Jones Senior Nurse Manager,
The Pembridge Palliative Care Centre

John Kapp User representative

Rosemary Lucey Clinical Support Co-ordinator,
Lynda Jackson Macmillan Centre

Dame Gill Oliver Director of Service Development,
Macmillan Cancer Relief

Jenny Penson Former Education Manager, North Devon Hospice

Dr David Peters Clinical Director, School of Integrated Health,
University of Westminster

Stephen Richards Head of Service Development,
London, Anglia, South East Region,
Macmillan Cancer Relief

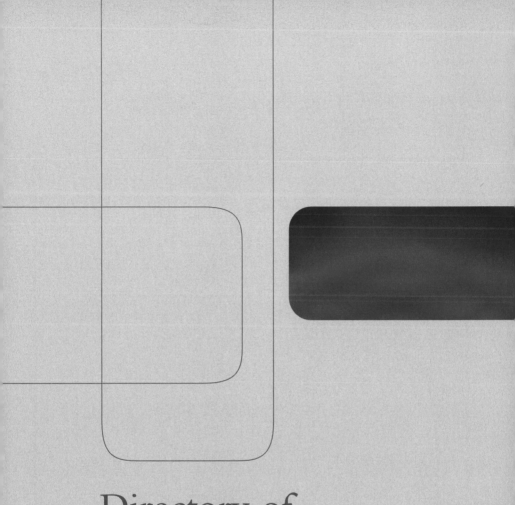

Directory of complementary therapy services

Locations of complementary therapy services in England and Wales

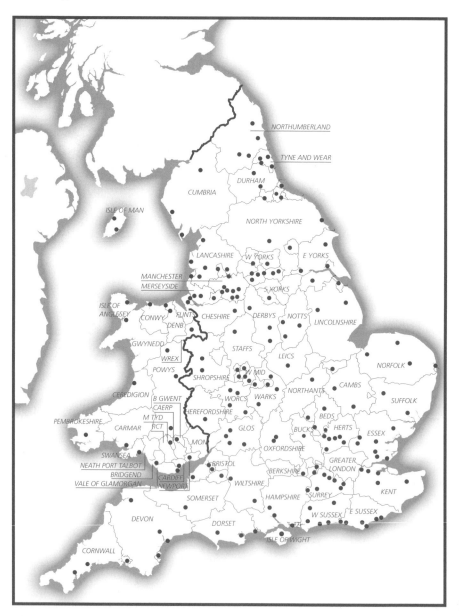

Locations of complementary therapy services in Scotland and Northern Ireland

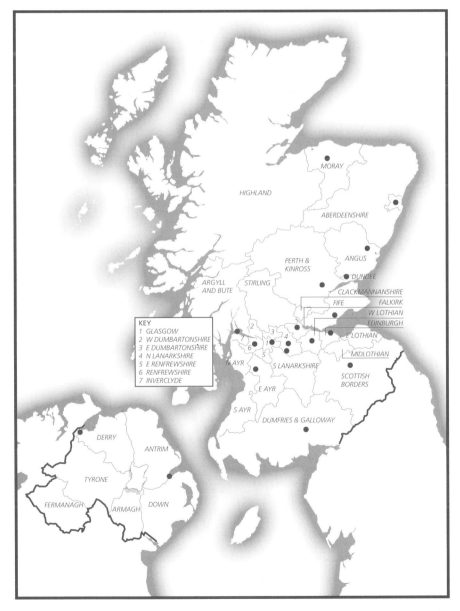

KEY
1 GLASGOW
2 W DUMBARTONSHIRE
3 E DUMBARTONSHIRE
4 N LANARKSHIRE
5 E RENFREWSHIRE
6 RENFREWSHIRE
7 INVERCLYDE

Locations of complementary therapy services in Greater London

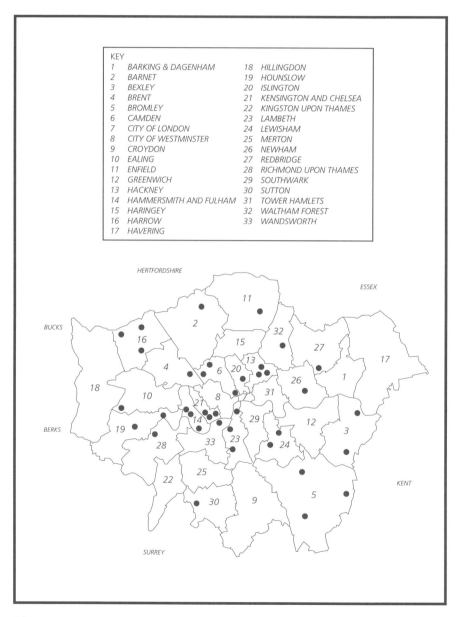

KEY
1	BARKING & DAGENHAM	18	HILLINGDON
2	BARNET	19	HOUNSLOW
3	BEXLEY	20	ISLINGTON
4	BRENT	21	KENSINGTON AND CHELSEA
5	BROMLEY	22	KINGSTON UPON THAMES
6	CAMDEN	23	LAMBETH
7	CITY OF LONDON	24	LEWISHAM
8	CITY OF WESTMINSTER	25	MERTON
9	CROYDON	26	NEWHAM
10	EALING	27	REDBRIDGE
11	ENFIELD	28	RICHMOND UPON THAMES
12	GREENWICH	29	SOUTHWARK
13	HACKNEY	30	SUTTON
14	HAMMERSMITH AND FULHAM	31	TOWER HAMLETS
15	HARINGEY	32	WALTHAM FOREST
16	HARROW	33	WANDSWORTH
17	HAVERING		

Index of county and Greater London maps

Full entries for all the complementary therapy services in the directory are detailed on the following pages. These are organised on a county-by-county basis, with the list of entries for each county being preceded in each case by a map for that county. The maps also show the nearby counties so you can refer to them if necessary.

Please note that the directory is organised alphabetically so services in the London and Manchester areas are listed under 'G' for Greater London and Greater Manchester and counties like West Sussex and East Yorkshire are listed under 'W' and 'E' respectively.

ENGLAND

INDEX OF MAPS

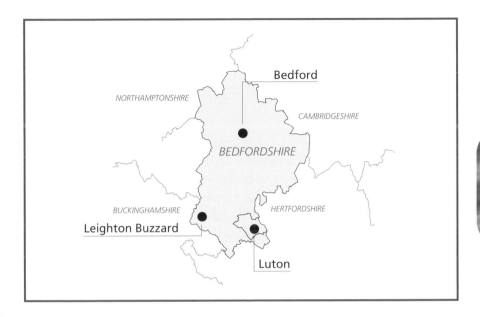

Complementary therapy services in

Bedfordshire

Bedford	• North Bedfordshire Day Care Hospice
	• Sue Ryder Care – St John's
Leighton Buzzard	• Health, Healing and Counselling Group
Luton	• Pasque Hospice

North Bedfordshire Day Care Hospice

Sue Nicholls, Senior Nurse   **01234 352015**
Gladys Ibbett House, 3 Linden Road, Bedford, Bedfordshire MK40 2DD

Day hospice

Therapies:	Art Therapy, Reflexology, Relaxation
Details:	Therapies available to clients on weekday mornings with Reflexology available to staff. Professional referral required for all therapies, which must also be booked in advance
Cost:	Charge may apply for Reflexology
Quality assurance:	Reflexologist checks medical history and consults with senior nurse. Checks for contra-indications. Consent form signed by patient and senior nurse. Patient condition/response assessed after each treatment and notes written up
Promotion:	Reflexology offered verbally to patients attending day care hospice. Patients referred for Reflexology by community Macmillan nurses

Sue Ryder Care – St John's

Myra Davies, Care Centre Manager   **01767 640622**
St John's Care Centre, St John's Road, Moggerhanger, Bedford, Bedfordshire MK44 3RJ

St John's is an 18-bed specialist palliative care centre that is part of the Sue Ryder Care network of care centres. Located in a rural setting, it offers short-term admissions for pain and symptom control, respite care and terminal care

Therapies:	Aromatherapy, Counselling, Massage, Meditation, Reflexology, Reiki, Relaxation, Spiritual Healing, Visualisation
Details:	All therapies are available to clients and staff on weekdays (9am-5pm), with counselling also available to carers. Outpatients may have timed appointments, inpatients receive

therapies as part of their care plan. All therapies are on a self-referral basis. Outpatients need to book in advance

Cost: All free of charge

Quality assurance: All staff fully trained in recognised certificated courses. Information leaflets provided for patients

Materials supplied: Range of supportive and teaching materials available

Promotion: Leaflets; posters; via care plan on admission; via care centre brochure

Health, Healing and Counselling Group

01525 373638

All Saints Church, Church Square, Leighton Buzzard, Bedfordshire LU7 7AE

The group aims to support people affected by life-threatening and chronic physical illness

Therapies: Acupuncture, Aromatherapy, Massage, Meditation, Reflexology, Reiki, Relaxation, Spiritual Healing, Visualisation

Details: Open Thursdays. Referral from medical/nursing staff or self-referral

Cost: There is a nominal £3 charge, but not being able to afford the fee does not exclude members from receiving a therapy

Quality assurance: All new members are asked to obtain GP's/specialist's consent using forms before receiving therapies

Materials supplied: Clients given relevant information by individual therapists

Promotion: Leaflets

Pasque Hospice

Mike Keel, Director of Nursing   **01582 492339**
Great Bramingham Lane, Luton, Bedfordshire LU3 3NT

Therapies:	Acupuncture, Aromatherapy, Art Therapy, Massage, Music Therapy, Reflexology, Relaxation, Shiatsu, Therapeutic Touch
Details:	Open weekdays providing therapies to clients with weekly Acupuncture sessions on Friday afternoons. Art Therapy is not available to carers. Self referral accepted for Art Therapy and Music Therapy; professional referral is required for Acupuncture, Aromatherapy, Massage, Reflexology, Relaxation, Shiatsu and Therapeutic Touch. Book in advance for Aromatherapy, Massage, Reflexology, Relaxation, Shiatsu and Therapeutic Touch
Cost:	All free of charge
Promotion:	In-house information

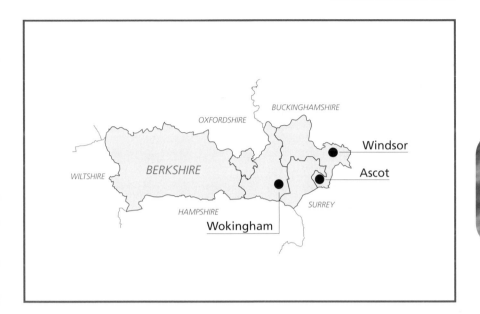

Complementary therapy services in
Berkshire

Ascot	• Paul Bevan Day Hospice
Windsor	• Thames Valley Hospice
Wokingham	• British Airways Macmillan House

Paul Bevan Day Hospice

Vivienne Shedden, Nurse Manager   **01344 877 877**
Paul Bevan House, Kings Ride, Ascot, Berkshire SL5 7RD

A day hospice run from a purpose-built unit

Therapies:	Aromatherapy, Art Therapy, Counselling, Hypnotherapy/Hypnosis, Massage, Music Therapy, Reflexology, Relaxation, Visualisation
Details:	Open weekdays except Thursday mornings with all therapies available to clients. Counselling is open to carers, and Aromatherapy, Counselling, Massage and Reflexology available to staff. All therapies on self referral except Hypnotherapy/Hypnosis requiring professional referral. Clients can be referred by healthcare professionals for Aromatherapy, Art Therapy, Massage, Music Therapy and Reflexology. Book in advance for Aromatherapy, Counselling, Massage, Reflexology
Cost:	All free of charge
Quality assurance:	Guidelines to practise in place. Therapists instructed by nursing staff. Patients told to check with medical advisers there are no contra-indications before starting therapy
Promotion:	Patient information leaflet; other care providers disseminate information

Thames Valley Hospice

Mandy Cutler, Complementary Therapist   **01753 842121**
Pine Lodge, Hatch Lane, Windsor, Berkshire SL4 3RW

Therapies:	Aromatherapy, Massage, Reflexology
Details:	Available to clients and staff on weekdays. Professional referral is required
Cost:	All free of charge
Quality assurance:	Medical referral to hospice details general medical condition. A complementary therapist completes an assessment for each

patient and discusses appropriate therapy. A complementary
therapist then completes a checklist to ensure there are no
contra-indications for particular therapy

Materials supplied: Relaxation tapes, introduction to therapies leaflet

Promotion: Hospice at home liaison team; hospice information booklet; other leaflets

British Airways Macmillan House

Annette Pembroke, Day Therapy Unit Nurse Manager   **0118 949 5029/5030**

Wokingham Hospital, Barkham Road, Wokingham, Berkshire RG41 2RE

A day therapy unit with a multidisciplinary team including Macmillan nurses

Therapies: Aromatherapy, Art Therapy, Massage, Relaxation, Nutritional Supplements

Details: All therapies are available to clients, with Aromatherapy and Massage open to carers and staff, and Relaxation open to carers. Advance booking is required for Aromatherapy, Art Therapy, Massage and Relaxation. Professional referral is required for all therapies. Aromatherapy is available weekdays except Thursdays; contact the unit for availability of other therapies

Cost: All free of charge although donations for treatment are accepted

Materials supplied: Leaflet on Aromatherapy

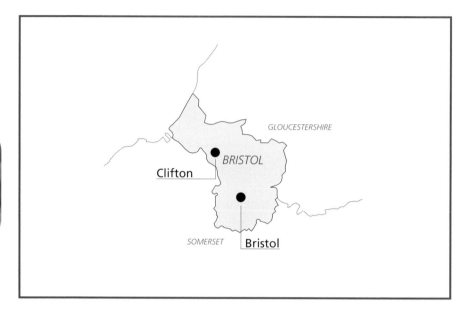

Complementary therapy services in

Bristol

Bristol	● Bristol Homeopathic Hospital
	● St Peter's Hospice
Clifton	● Bristol Cancer Help Centre

Bristol Homeopathic Hospital

Elizabeth Thompson, Consultant Homeopathic Physician   **0117 973 1231**

Cotham Hill, Bristol BS6 6PD

Outpatient department with access to 5 inpatient beds

Therapies:	Homeopathy, Iscador
Details:	Open to clients on Tuesday afternoons and Wednesday mornings. Self referral accepted for Iscador with Homeopathy requiring professional referral
Cost:	All free of charge
Quality assurance:	Doctor-led service with integration of understanding of clinical condition. Leaflets available on side effects of Homeopathy and Iscador
Promotion:	Word of mouth

St Peter's Hospice

Dr D Spence, Consultant in Palliative Medicine   **0117 915 9225 (Brentry)**
                                                             0117 915 9262 (Knowle)

Charlton Road, Brentry, Bristol BS10 6NL

St Peter's is on two sites in Bristol: Charlton Road, Brentry and St Agnes Ave, Knowle

Therapies:	Acupuncture, Aromatherapy, Massage, Music Therapy, Reflexology, Relaxation, Shiatsu
Details:	Therapies are provided by volunteers to patients attending the day hospice or admitted to the inpatient unit, with Massage additionally available to carers. A volunteer should be present in both day hospices and in both inpatient units every day, but this is not always possible
Cost:	All free of charge
Quality assurance:	The therapist is given information on patient's condition by health professional and then offers a service to the patient who may accept or decline. The therapist is warned about

	body areas not to touch (eg. lymphoedemous limbs, radiation burns)
Promotion:	Welcome book on inpatient unit mentions complementary therapies; nurses in day hospice advise patients of availability; community nurses mention therapies available; patient information leaflets currently being written

Bristol Cancer Help Centre

Telephone help line 0117 980 9505

Grove House, Cornwallis Grove, Clifton, Bristol BS8 4PG

The Help Centre operates a residential therapy programme for those with cancer and their supporters, as well as workshops and courses for healthcare professionals and carers

Therapies:	Art Therapy, Counselling, Massage, Meditation, Music Therapy, Nutritional Programmes, Nutritional Supplements, Relaxation, Shiatsu, Spiritual Healing, Visualisation
Details:	All therapies are available to clients and carers with Meditation and Spiritual Healing open to staff. Self referral is accepted for all therapies. Open weekdays (and sometimes weekday evenings). Book in advance for all therapies except Spiritual Healing, which is available to drop-in clients
Cost:	Fees are charged for all therapies
Quality assurance:	Take history of patient's condition and past medical history. Doctor's consultation to check for possible interactions
Materials supplied:	Videos, cassettes, literature
Promotion:	Through the media; literature; website (www.bristolcancerhelp.org); telephone services

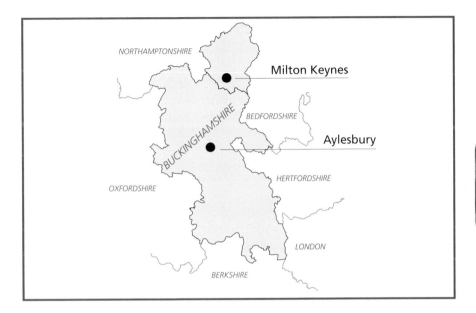

Complementary therapy services in

Buckinghamshire

Aylesbury	• Stoke Mandeville Hospital NHS Trust
Milton Keynes	• Milton Keynes Cancer Support Group
	• Willen Hospice

Stoke Mandeville Hospital NHS Trust

Sister June Wilson   **01296 315120**

Cancer Care & Haematology Unit, Mandeville Road, Aylesbury, Buckinghamshire
HP21 8AL

The Cancer Care & Chemotherapy/Haematology Unit is a purpose-built day unit.
There is a designated area for complementary therapies. All volunteers are mature,
trained, female therapists. The complementary therapy service is free at the point of
delivery

Therapies:	Aromatherapy, Massage, Reflexology, Therapeutic Touch
Details:	Open on weekday mornings and all day Tuesdays for clients with therapies available to carers if time allows. Self referral is accepted for all therapies (can be referred by healthcare professional). Advance booking is required
Cost:	All free of charge
Quality assurance:	Particular therapy recommended by nursing staff. Full consultation before therapy is given
Promotion:	Recommendation from nursing and medical staff; posters; word of mouth from other patients

Milton Keynes Cancer Support Group

Peter or Wendy   **01908 375694/606602**

24 Springfield Court, Ravensbourne Place, Springfield, Milton Keynes,
Buckinghamshire MK6 3JJ

Therapies:	Counselling, Meditation, Reiki, Relaxation, Spiritual Healing, Visualisation
Details:	Available to clients on request for one-hour sessions only. Self referral accepted for all therapies
Cost:	All free of charge
Quality assurance:	Know the patients and helpers well
Materials supplied:	CDs
Promotion:	Word-of-mouth recommendations

Willen Hospice

Mrs Jenni Acres, Director of Nursing　　　　　　　　**0190 8663 636**

Manor Farm, Milton Road, Milton Keynes, Buckinghamshire MK15 9AB

Therapies:	Aromatherapy, Massage, Reflexology
Details:	All therapies must be booked in advance; appointments with clients are booked to meet patients' needs and are influenced by availability of therapists as most are volunteers. Professional referrals are required. Aromatherapy and Massage are available to staff
Cost:	All free of charge
Promotion:	Introduced by clinical nurse specialists. Information leaflets

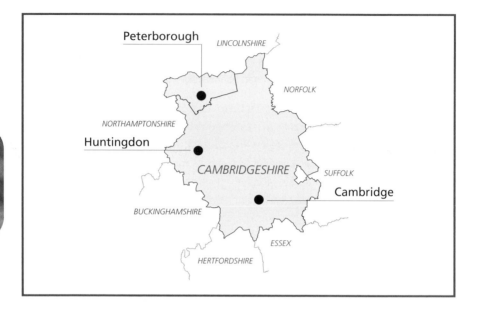

Complementary therapy services in

Cambridgeshire

Cambridge
- Addenbrooke's Hospital
- Arthur Rank Hospice
- Cambridge Cancer Help Centre
- East Anglia's Children's Hospices

Huntingdon
- Hinchingbrooke Healthcare NHS Trust

Peterborough
- Sue Ryder Care Centre - Thorpe Hall
- The Robert Horrell Day Centre

Addenbrooke's Hospital

Carole Chilverton, Senior Macmillan Nurse   **01223 274404**
Box 193, Oncology Department, Hills Road, Cambridge, Cambridgeshire CB2 2QQ

Therapies:	Meditation, Relaxation, Visualisation
Details:	Therapies are available on wards as appropriate to treatment, with all therapies also available to carers and staff. Professional referral is required
Cost:	All free of charge
Quality assurance:	After full assessment of patient's needs, Relaxation will be offered as part of treatment. Carers meet the same criteria. Practitioner is trained in depth in Relaxation
Materials supplied:	Leaflets on Relaxation are being developed

Arthur Rank Hospice

Angela Chisholm or Anne Barnes or Mary Smith   **01223 723140**
Brookfields Hospital, 351 Mill Road, Cambridge, Cambridgeshire CB1 3DF

Complementary therapists work in day therapy and in the hospice. They also treat carers and a few outpatients

Therapies:	Aromatherapy, Counselling, Massage, Reflexology, Reiki, Relaxation, Visualisation
Details:	Open weekdays except Monday mornings. Offers all therapies to clients and carers, with Counselling available to staff. Professional referral is required for Counselling only. Drop-in available for all therapies. Book in advance for Aromatherapy, Counselling, Massage and Reflexology
Cost:	All free of charge. Nutritional advice is given
Quality assurance:	Understanding of patient's condition. GP's consent required for day therapy patients. Information provided on side effects of treatment
Materials supplied:	Literature, cassettes and verbal advice
Promotion:	Leaflets and posters

Cambridge Cancer Help Centre

Ann Dingley, Co-ordinator   **01223 566151**
1A Stockwell Street, off Mill Road, Cambridge, Cambridgeshire CB1 3ND

The centre is a very informal and friendly support group comprised of ordinary people, some of whom have or have had cancer or who are caring for or have cared for someone who has or who has had cancer

Therapies:	Art Therapy, Counselling, Meditation, Music Therapy, Reiki, Relaxation, Spiritual Healing, Visualisation
Details:	Offers all therapies to clients, carers and staff on Tuesday mornings and Wednesday mornings only. Self referrals are accepted. Therapies except Counselling are available on a drop-in basis; Counselling requires advance booking
Cost:	For Counselling, a donation is welcome for the centre's funds
Quality assurance:	The counsellors and healers are responsible for this
Materials supplied:	Help with accessing information; Bristol Cancer Help Centre video; library; information about Homeopathic Hospital, Macmillan, other support groups, etc

East Anglia's Children's Hospices

Mrs Alex South, Head of Care   **01223 860306**
Church Lane, Milton, Cambridge, Cambridgeshire CB4 6AB

Comprising three children's hospices across East Anglia, providing a service to children and young people with life-limiting/threatening conditions. The Hospices also offer care in the community

Therapies:	Art Therapy, Drama Therapy, Massage, Music Therapy, Nutritional Programmes, Relaxation, Nutritional Supplements
Details:	Available as required (no referral or booking necessary).

Treatment is individualised for each child. All complementary therapies are offered to children as part of their routine care

Cost: All free of charge

Promotion: Letters to children's parents

Hinchingbrooke Healthcare NHS Trust

Heather Sawyer, Macmillan Clinical Services Manager   **01840 416103**

Hinchingbrooke Hospital, Hinchingbrooke Park, Huntingdon, Cambridgeshire PE29 6NT

Hinchingbrooke operates a palliative care team working in both hospital and community settings

Therapies: Aromatherapy, Massage

Details: Open Mondays to clients only. Requires professional referral and advance booking

Cost: Fee charged where possible

Quality assurance: Patients thoroughly assessed prior to therapy commencing. Therapists are all trained nurses

Materials supplied: Booklets

Promotion: Leaflet; via Macmillan nurses/chemotherapy staff

Sue Ryder Care Centre – Thorpe Hall

Bruce Wringe, Acting Care Centre Manager   **01733 330060**

Thorpe Hall, Longthorpe, Peterborough, Cambridgeshire PE3 6LW

A 22-bedded specialist palliative care inpatient unit providing symptom management, physical, emotional, psychological and spiritual care. The day centre has 12 places a day for those with neurological conditions

Therapies: Aromatherapy, Massage, Reflexology, Reiki, Shiatsu, Spiritual Healing, Nutritional Supplements

Details:	All therapies are available to clients, with Aromatherapy, Massage, Reflexology, Reiki and Spiritual Healing therapies also available to staff. Professional referral and advance booking required. (Please contact for details of opening/availability.)
Cost:	Free of charge to clients, with staff charged at a reduced rate
Promotion:	Via hospice brochure; via information leaflet; via community and hospital Macmillan nurses; via hospice liaison sister; via nurses and doctors

The Robert Horrell Day Centre

Robert Horrell Macmillan Centre   **01733 875114**
Edith Cavell Hospital, Bretton Gate, Peterborough, Cambridgeshire PE3 9GZ

The Macmillan Centre provides day care and outpatient services

Therapies:	Aromatherapy, Art Therapy, Massage, Reflexology, Reiki, Relaxation, Nutritional Supplements
Details:	Open on Mondays and Tuesday, Wednesday and Thursday mornings. Requires professional referral for all therapies except Art Therapy which requires advance booking
Cost:	Free of charge
Quality assurance:	Information on side effects of treatment available. Patient's treatment fully understood and reiterated before treatment commences
Materials supplied:	Day Centre leaflets, CancerBACUP's, nutritional; cassettes for relaxation
Promotion:	Leaflet; part of the oncology assessment form

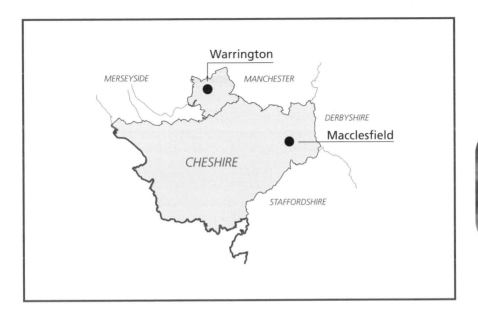

Complementary therapy services in

Cheshire

Macclesfield	● East Cheshire Hospice
Warrington	● St Rocco's Hospice
	● Warrington District Hospital

East Cheshire Hospice

Leslie Thompson, Matron   **01625 610364**

Millbank Drive, Macclesfield, Cheshire SK10 3DR

Therapies:	Acupuncture, Aromatherapy, Art Therapy, Counselling, Hypnotherapy/Hypnosis, Massage, Reflexology, Reiki, Relaxation, Therapeutic Touch, Visualisation
Details:	Open weekdays to clients, with Aromatherapy, Art Therapy, Counselling, Massage, Reflexology, Reiki, Relaxation, Therapeutic Touch, Visualisation available to carers, and Aromatherapy, Counselling, Massage, Reflexology, Therapeutic Touch available to staff. Professional referral and advance booking are required
Cost:	All free of charge
Quality assurance:	Patients are referred through GP or medical/surgical team. Individual therapists decide with patients which therapies are appropriate. Therapist has guidelines: suitability depends on patient condition and any treatments being received. Assessments made prior to commencement of treatment
Materials supplied:	Basic literature regarding therapies
Promotion:	Supplies the following healthcare professionals with information packs and referral forms – primary healthcare team, specialist nurses e.g. Macmillan nurses and palliative care consultant

St Rocco's Hospice

Elizabeth Eccles, Matron   **01925 575780**

Lockton Lane, Bewsey, Warrington, Cheshire WA5 0BW

Therapies:	Acupuncture, Aromatherapy, Art Therapy, Massage, Meditation, Reflexology, Reiki, Relaxation, Spiritual Healing, Nutritional Supplements, Therapeutic Touch
Details:	Open weekdays and Friday mornings to clients and carers,

with Aromatherapy, Massage, Reflexology, Reiki, Spiritual Healing and Therapeutic Touch available to staff. Professional referral is required and advance booking is available. (Drop in for Aromatherapy, Art Therapy, Massage, Meditation, Reflexology, Relaxation, Spiritual Healing, Nutritional Supplements, Therapeutic Touch.)

Cost: All free of charge

Quality assurance: All complementary therapies given by doctor, hospice's physiotherapist or member of nursing staff with diploma in relevant complementary therapy. Many staff nurses have been seconded to do diplomas in Aromatherapy or Reflexology. Some staff nurses do day care sessions as a therapist

Materials supplied: Hospice video

Promotion: Leaflets; hospice video made with patients and carers in mind; brochures; hospice 'pack'; using weekly Warrington Guardian newspaper

Warrington District Hospital

Clare Inman

Palliative Care, Lovely Lane, Warrington, Cheshire WA5 1QG

At present, nobody at this hospital offers complementary therapies to patients. Complementary therapies are available for staff with health problems

Therapies: Aromatherapy, Reflexology, Reiki

Details: Serves only hospital staff on professional referral

Cost: Free of charge

Quality assurance: Has to be medically indicated – staff must have a health problem according to set criteria to be put forward for complementary therapies

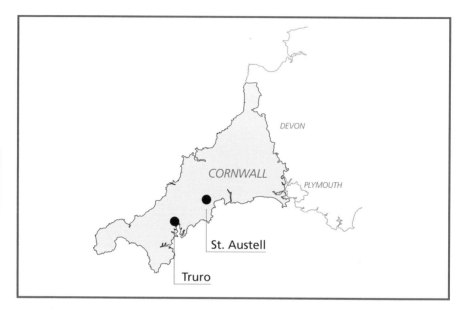

Complementary therapy services in
Cornwall

St. Austell   • Mount Edgcumbe Hospice
Truro   • Cornwall Cancer Help Groups (Truro)
                         • Cornwall Macmillan Service

Mount Edgcumbe Hospice

Wendy Leach, Complementary Therapy Co-ordinator   **01726 65711**

Porthpean Road, St. Austell, Cornwall PL26 6AB

Mount Edgcumbe is a hospice setting with an inpatient ward and a day care service

Therapies:	Aromatherapy, Art Therapy, Massage, Music Therapy, Reiki, Relaxation, Visualisation
Details:	Open Tuesday to Thursday, with therapies available on the ward on Mondays, Wednesdays and Fridays (08.30 to 17.30). Staff may receive Massage on Friday evenings. Massage and Relaxation therapies are open to staff and carers, with Aromatherapy and Reiki additionally available to carers. Advance booking is required for Aromatherapy, Massage, Reiki and Relaxation. Clients can be referred for CTs by health professionals. Self referrals are accepted for Aromatherapy, Massage and Reiki.
Cost:	Please enquire
Quality assurance:	Guidelines for all therapies practised. Guidelines for therapist self-care. Complementary therapy policy. Standards on all therapies practised – reviewed annually
Materials supplied:	CDs and tapes for relaxation, CancerBACUP literature, information on complementary and alternative therapies
Promotion:	Welcome leaflet; information leaflet given to all GPs; talks to local Mermaid Centre; talks and lectures to English Nursing Board groups, nursing homes, volunteers, GP trainees; demonstrations to COPD groups through day care

Cornwall Cancer Help Groups (Truro)

Miss M Langridge, Secretary   **01872 272652**
2 Crescent Rise, Truro, Cornwall TR1 3ER

The Help Groups meet fortnightly at Copeland Court, a former convent, on the edge of Truro. From January 2002, they are scheduled to hold some sessions in the oncology department of Treliske Hospital

Therapies:	Meditation, Reiki, Relaxation, Spiritual Healing, T'ai Chi, Visualisation
Details:	Therapies are available to clients, carers and staff twice a month on Thursdays (10.30–12.00). Self referral is accepted for all therapies
Cost:	All free of charge
Quality assurance:	All therapists are registered healers
Materials supplied:	Information about Bristol Cancer Help Centre, Cancerlink and CancerBACUP
Promotion:	Leaflets; posters; talks to interested groups through contacts within the hospital service

Cornwall Macmillan Service

Rosie Hays   **01872 354383**
3 St Clement Vean, Tregolls Road, Truro, Cornwall TR1 1RN

Therapies:	Aromatherapy, Massage, Reflexology, Relaxation
Details:	Therapies are available to clients on Tuesday, Wednesday and Thursday mornings with Reflexology also available at home on Tuesday evenings. Professional referral is required
Cost:	All free of charge
Quality assurance:	Referral guidelines; referral form from nurse; GP approval
Promotion:	Through day care attendance; via Macmillan nurses

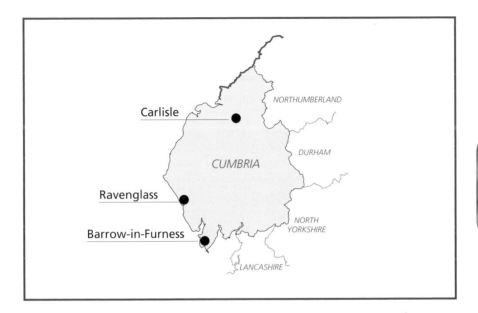

Complementary therapy services in

Cumbria

Barrow-In-Furness	• Furness Cancer Support Group
Carlisle	• Eden Valley Hospice
	• North Cumbria Acute Hospitals NHS Trust
Ravenglass	• Centre for Complementary Care

Furness Cancer Support Group

Anne or Elaine   **01229 471650 / 834016**
Atkinson Health Centre, Barrow-In-Furness, Cumbria

Therapies:	Aromatherapy, Indian Head (& Neck) Massage, Reflexology, Reiki, Relaxation
Details:	Available on Wednesday afternoons with Aromatherapy available on Fridays by appointment. All therapies are available to clients (and to carers/staff with the exception of Aromatherapy). Professional referral is only required for Aromatherapy, which also requires advance booking
Cost:	All free of charge
Quality assurance:	GP signs consent form. For Aromatherapy, clients are referred by Macmillan or lymphoedema nurses
Promotion:	Leaflets and posters; talking to new clients

Eden Valley Hospice

Heather King, Practice Development Nurse   **01228 817625**
Durdar Road, Carlisle, Cumbria CA2 4SD

Eden Valley is an independent hospice established 10 years ago

Therapies:	Aromatherapy, Art Therapy, Massage, Reflexology, Reiki, Relaxation, Nutritional Supplements, Visualisation
Details:	A team of nurses provides the majority of therapies, so it is possible to offer therapies to clients at all times except for holiday periods. Additionally, Aromatherapy, Massage,

Reflexology and Reiki are available to carers and staff. All therapies require advance booking, with only Aromatherapy, Massage and Reflexology needing professional referral

Cost: All free of charge

Quality assurance: All nurse therapies take a full patient history. If patient has self-referred then consent is requested from either hospice medical staff or patient's GP

Materials supplied: General information which nurses have gathered from courses/conferences

Promotion: Leaflets; patient information books

North Cumbria Acute Hospitals NHS Trust

Mrs Claire Huddart, Cancer Services Manager   **01228 523444**

The Cumberland Infirmary, New Town Road, Carlisle, Cumbria CA2 7HY

Therapies: Aromatherapy, Massage, Reiki

Details: Therapies are available on Tuesday mornings to clients, with Aromatherapy also available to staff. All require advance booking but not professional referral

Book in advance: All therapies

Cost: All free of charge

Quality assurance: Medical colleagues in the hospital and community are made aware of procedures that clients are undergoing in accordance with the written policy. Potential problems are discussed prior to the start of the therapy

Promotion: Leaflets; word of mouth

Centre for Complementary Care

Gretchen Stevens, Director **01229 717355**

Knott End, Birkby Road, Ravenglass, Cumbria CA18 1RT

The Centre provides peace and healing in the beautiful and secluded Eskdale valley. It offers support, information and treatment for relief of sickness, pain, fear and sorrow

Therapies:	Spiritual Healing
Details:	Therapies are available to clients every weekday on advance booking and self referral
Cost:	Therapies free of charge, but donation appreciated
Quality assurance:	We offer healing by gentle touch, which is suitable for all ages and all conditions
Materials supplied:	Library available to clients
Promotion:	Quarterly newsletters; feature coverage in local and national press, radio and TV; publication of research data; word of mouth

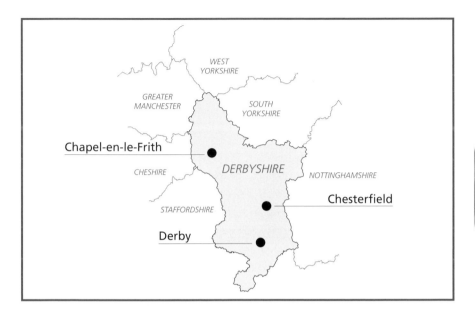

Complementary therapy services in

Derbyshire

Chapel-en-le-Frith	• Blythe House Day Care Hospice
Chesterfield	• Chesterfield and North Derbyshire Royal Hospital
Derby	• Derbyshire Royal Infirmary
	• Treetops Hospice

Blythe House Day Care Hospice

Hazel Larman, Nurse Manager   **01298 815388**

Blythe House, Eccles Fold Road, High Peak, Chapel-en-le-Frith, Derbyshire SK23 9TJ

The hospice operates from a purpose-built day centre. The day care service includes complementary therapies which are offered for five hours a day, three days a week

Therapies:	Aromatherapy, Art Therapy, Massage, Indian Head (& Neck) Massage, Reflexology, Reiki, Relaxation, Visualisation
Details:	All therapies are available to clients from Tuesday to Thursday with a drop-in service available on Mondays. Aromatherapy, Massage, Reiki, Relaxation and Visualisation are also available to carers. No professional referral is required (but clients can be referred for CTs via healthcare professionals). Visualisation requires advance booking
Cost:	All free of charge
Materials supplied:	Explanatory leaflet about therapies given to clients
Promotion:	Day care leaflets given to patients, carers, GPs, Macmillan and district nurses

Chesterfield and North Derbyshire Royal Hospital

Dr David Brooks   **01246 277271 x 2693**

Calow, Chesterfield, Derbyshire S44 5BL

Therapies:	Acupuncture, Hypnotherapy/Hypnosis, Relaxation
Details:	Available on Tuesday afternoons to clients on professional referral
Cost:	All free of charge
Quality assurance:	Part of assessment that takes place in outpatient clinic
Promotion:	Discuss during outpatient clinic

Derbyshire Royal Infirmary

Kerry Pape, Senior Nurse Cancer Services   **01332 347141 x4266**
London Road, Derby, Derbyshire DE1 2QY

The Infirmary's cancer service includes oncology, haematology and specialist palliative medicine

Therapies: Massage, Reflexology, Relaxation
Details: Therapies are available to clients on Mondays and Thursdays on professional referral
Cost: All free of charge
Quality assurance: Discussion with complementary therapist at multidisciplinary team meeting
Promotion: Referred from specialist palliative care team, including community

Treetops Hospice

Anne Richards, Nurse Manager   **0115 949 1264**
Derby Road, Risley, Derby, Derbyshire DE72 3SS

Therapies: Aromatherapy, Massage, Reflexology, Reiki, Relaxation
Details: Therapies are available to clients and carers on Wednesdays. Professional referral is required for Aromatherapy, Massage, Reflexology and Reiki. All therapies require advance booking
Cost: All free of charge
Quality assurance: GP's advice and consent sought for every referral. Guidelines on appropriate use of therapy and contra-indications.Post-treatment advice leaflet for clients. Full medical history taken on first visit
Promotion: Leaflets; word of mouth; newsletters

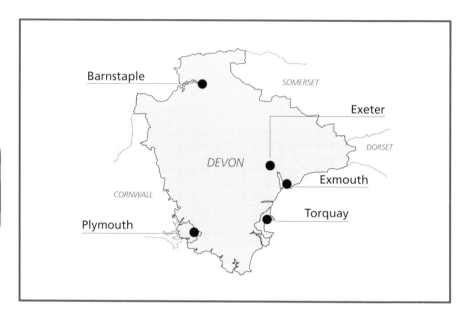

Complementary therapy services in

Devon

Barnstaple	• North Devon Hospice
Exeter	• Cancer Support and Information Centre (Exeter)
Exmouth	• The Quiet Mind Centre
Plymouth	• Mustard Tree Macmillan Centre
	• St. Luke's Hospice
Torquay	• CanCope
	• Rowcroft – Torbay & South Devon Hospice

North Devon Hospice

Mr Richard Kane, Director of Nursing   **01271 344248**
Deer Park Road, Newport, Barnstaple, Devon EX32 0HU

Therapies:	Acupuncture, Aromatherapy, Counselling, Massage, Nutritional Programmes, Reflexology, Spiritual Healing
Details:	All therapies are available Monday to Saturday, to clients and carers, with Counselling open to staff. Professional referral is required for all therapies
Cost:	All free of charge
Quality assurance:	Complementary therapy operational policy
Materials supplied:	Information leaflets
Promotion:	Leaflets; word of mouth

Cancer Support and Information Centre (Exeter)

Anne Clemo, Complementary Therapy Co-ordinator   **01392 402086**
Medical Outpatients, Area B, Royal Devon & Exeter Health Care NHST, Barrack Road, Exeter, Devon EX2 5DW

A cancer support and information service for people whose lives are affected by cancer. It is based in the medical outpatient department of the Royal Devon & Exeter Hospital at Wonford

Therapies:	Aromatherapy, Massage, Reflexology, Relaxation
Details:	Therapies are available to clients and carers on Mondays (16.30 – 18.30) and Thursdays (13.30 – 19.00). Advance booking is required for Aromatherapy, Massage and Reflexology. Self referrals are accepted
Cost:	All free of charge
Quality assurance:	Contra-indications checklist. Assessment by therapist
Materials supplied:	Healthy Living Sheets
Promotion:	Leaflets; posters on wards; nurses and doctors inform patients

The Quiet Mind Centre

Mrs Bobby Neil, General Manager　　　　　　　　　　**01395 270070**
10a Salterton Road, Exmouth, Devon EX8 2BW

A voluntary organisation that helps anyone, including those affected by cancer, with any stress-related, physical or emotional problem and who is on benefits, a pension or low income

Therapies:	Alexander Technique, Aromatherapy, Counselling, Homeopathy, Massage, Meditation, Osteopathy, Reflexology, Reiki, Relaxation, Shiatsu, Spiritual Healing, Nutritional Supplements, Visualisation
Details:	Therapies are available on weekdays to clients and carers through self referral. Advance booking necessary for all therapies (clients can be referred by health professional for Alexander Technique)
Cost:	Free of charge but donations are welcome
Promotion:	Leaflets; newsletters; word of mouth

Mustard Tree Macmillan Centre

Pat Stapleton　　　　　　　　　　　　　　　　　　**01752 763672**
Level 3, Derriford Hospital, Plymouth, Devon PL6 8DH

The Mustard Tree Centre operates within a purpose-built information and support centre adjacent to the oncology centre

Therapies:	Aromatherapy, Counselling, Cranio-Sacral Therapy, Massage, Meditation, Reflexology, Reiki, Relaxation, Spiritual Healing
Details:	All therapies are open to clients and carers on weekdays. Self referrals are accepted on all therapies with drop in available on Counselling, Meditation and Relaxation. Advance booking is necessary for Aromatherapy, Cranio-Sacral Therapy, Massage,

Reflexology, Reiki and Spiritual Healing. Clients can be referred by health professionals for Counselling

Cost: All free of charge

Quality assurance: Although patients can self-refer for complementary therapies, suitability is often discussed with clinician. Full history taken before treatment commences. Protocol for therapies in place

Materials supplied: Contra-indications checklist and after-care advice

Promotion: Booklet; recommendations from clinicians and other staff; lectures to staff who, in turn, inform patients

St Luke's Hospice

Helen Frances, Complementary Therapy Co-ordinator   **01752 401 172**

Stamford Road, Turnchapel, Plymouth, Devon PL9 9XA

Therapies: Acupuncture, Aromatherapy, Homeopathy, Massage, Indian Head (& Neck) Massage, Osteopathy, Reflexology, Reiki, Therapeutic Touch

Details: Therapies are available to clients on weekdays through professional referral

Cost: All free of charge

Quality assurance: Protocol and procedures for referral. Referrals made via complementary therapy co-ordinator for allocation to therapists. Therapists have access to patient notes and can discuss any concerns with doctor, nurse, etc

Materials supplied: Information booklet for patients recently developed

Promotion: Complementary therapy booklet outlining all therapies provided. Information provided from complementary therapy service to doctors, nurses, etc

CanCope

Ian Collins, Treasurer or Maggie Bose, Chairman	**01803 312098**
	or 01803 328689

First Floor, 20 Tor Hill Road, Torquay, Devon TQ2 5RD

The CanCope facility is a support centre which amongst other services offers complementary therapies

Therapies:	Autogenic Training, Counselling, Cranio-Sacral Therapy, Reflexology, Relaxation, Visualisation
Details:	Therapies are by appointment at a mutually convenient time to both clients and carers on self referral (clients may be referred by health professionals for Counselling). All therapies can be booked in advance with drop-in available for Reflexology.
Cost:	All free of charge
Materials supplied:	Literature on different complementary therapies is available for clients to consult
Promotion:	Leaflets; posters; word of mouth

Rowcroft – Torbay & South Devon Hospice

Liz Westwood	**01803 210800**

Rowcroft House, Avenue Road, Torquay, Devon TQ2 5LS

An 18-bedded specialist palliative care unit plus Macmillan community team operating a hospice-at-home service. Complementary therapies are provided in hospice but a multidisciplinary team visit patients in the community or provides an outpatient service

Therapies:	Aromatherapy, Counselling, Massage, Meditation, Music Therapy, Reflexology, Relaxation, Visualisation
Details:	Available weekdays to clients (Aromatherapy, Counselling, Massage, Music Therapy, Reflexology, Relaxation and

Visualisation); carers (Aromatherapy, Counselling, Massage, Music Therapy, Reflexology and Relaxation) and staff (Aromatherapy, Counselling, Massage, Meditation, Music Therapy, Reflexology and Relaxation). All therapies are available on self-referral and require advance booking

Cost: All free of charge

Quality assurance: Self-referral but in agreement with GP. Macmillan nurse input

Promotion: Patient leaflets; flyers; patient handbook

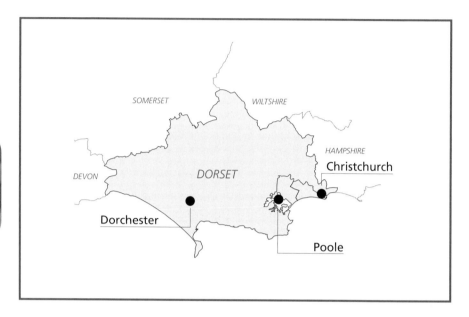

Complementary therapy services in

Dorset

Christchurch	● Christchurch Hospital
Dorchester	● CancerCare Dorset
Poole	● Poole Hospital

Christchurch Hospital

Heather Rogers   **01202 705291**
Macmillan Unit, Fairmile Road, Christchurch, Dorset

Christchurch Hospital is an NHS palliative care unit consisting of a 20-bedded
inpatient unit, six palliative care sisters, a hospital-based palliative care nurse specialist
and a day centre

Therapies:	Aromatherapy, Counselling, Massage
Details:	Therapies are available all week (including evenings) to clients and staff, with Aromatherapy and Counselling also available to carers. Professional referral and advance booking are necessary
Cost:	All free of charge
Quality assurance:	Discussion between aromatherapists and medical team
Materials supplied:	Aromatherapist supplies details
Promotion:	In the ward information leaflet

CancerCare Dorset

Gillian Walsham, Director of Nursing   **01305 269898**
The Undercroft, Herringston Road, Dorchester, Dorset DT1 2SJ

CancerCare provides specialist nurses who work in the community to advise, inform
and support patients as soon as cancer is diagnosed. It also has volunteers and runs a
bereavement support service. All complementary therapies are given in clients' homes
by arrangement

Therapies:	Aromatherapy, Massage
Details:	All treatments are given in clients' homes on professional referral and by arrangement with the therapists. Therapies are also available to carers and staff
Cost:	All free of charge. A charge is usually made after the first three sessions. Complementary therapies are also offered to the bereaved and an 'Aromatherapy at Home' service is being piloted

Quality assurance:	Policies, guidelines and protocols; referral criteria. Specialist nurse qualified in complementary healthcare reviews all referrals. Assessment of patient/client recorded prior to treatment by therapist. Referring nurse provides information on patient's condition and state of health
Materials supplied:	Information leaflets and booklet; contact number for advice/help
Promotion:	Information booklet and leaflets; nurses inform patients/carers who may benefit; specialist nurse referral. Bereavement workers inform clients who may benefit

Poole Hospital

Jenny Vestey   **01202 448268**
Oncology Directorate, Longfleet Road, Poole, Dorset BH15 2JB

Poole Hospital's oncology directorate includes the Forest Holme Hospice and constitutes part of the Dorset Cancer Centre

Therapies:	Aromatherapy, Counselling, Massage, Meditation, Reflexology, Relaxation, Visualisation, Yoga
Details:	Available to clients from Monday to Wednesday, with Counselling and Massage available to staff and Counselling open to carers. Self referrals are accepted for all therapies and all but Aromatherapy must be booked in advance
Cost:	Free of charge for Aromatherapy, Counselling, Reflexology, Relaxation, Visualisation and Yoga. A fee is payable for Massage
Quality assurance:	No written procedure – therapist liaises with consultants
Materials supplied:	Patient information pack
Promotion:	Patient information pack; individual leaflets; word of mouth by all staff

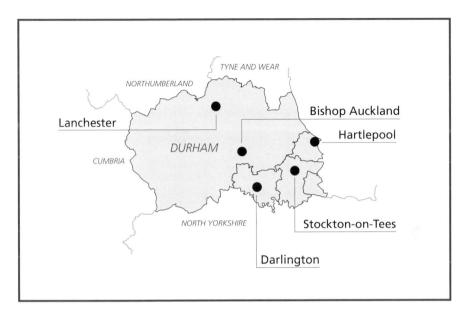

Complementary therapy services in

Durham

Bishop Auckland	• Butterwick Hospice
Darlington	• Coping with Cancer Darlington & District
	• South Durham Healthcare NHS Trust
Hartlepool	• Hartlepool and District Hospice
Lanchester	• Willow Burn Hospice
Stockton-on-Tees	• Butterwick Hospice & Butterwick House Children's Hospice

Butterwick Hospice

Gwynn Featonby, (Butterwick Hospice, Stockton)   **01642 607742**
Macmillan House, Woodhouse Lane, Bishop Auckland, Durham DL14 6JU

The hospice provides day hospice care on Wednesday, Thursday and Friday

Therapies:	Acupuncture, Aromatherapy, Relaxation
Details:	Therapies are available to clients from Wednesday to Friday. Self referrals are accepted for Aromatherapy and Relaxation with Acupuncture requiring professional referral. Clients can be referred through healthcare professional for Relaxation
Cost:	All free of charge
Quality assurance:	Assessed by doctor. Qualified aromatherapist is aware of side effects and contra-indications to the use of some oils. Qualified physiotherapist practises Acupuncture
Promotion:	Following referral for day care; through community and hospital staff; day care leaflets

Coping with Cancer Darlington & District

Jane Bradshaw, Hospice Director   **01325 254321**
St Teresa's Hospice, The Woodlands, 91 Woodland Road, Darlington, Durham DL3 7UA

Therapies:	Acupuncture, Aromatherapy, Counselling, Massage, Reflexology, Reiki, Relaxation, Nutritional Supplements
Details:	Therapies are available to clients on weekdays and Tuesday evenings monthly. Additionally, Counselling, Massage and Relaxation are available to carers and staff. Professional referral is only necessary for Nutritional Supplements. All therapies except Counselling and Massage need to be booked in advance

Cost:	All free of charge
Quality assurance:	Information on contra-indications of treatments. Notes available to appropriate professionals/therapists. Clients' consent obtained
Materials supplied:	Cassettes, booklets
Promotion:	Leaflets; posters; recommendations; referrals from other agencies

South Durham Healthcare NHS Trust

Lorraine Legg, Lead Nurse for Cancer Services   **01325 743027**
Memorial Hospital, Hollyhurst Road, Darlington, Durham DL3 6HX

The trust provides hospital and community healthcare to people in South Durham and parts of North Yorkshire. It cares for patients in seven hospitals, 15 health centres and in various clinics, as well as in patients' own homes

Therapies:	Acupuncture, Aromatherapy, Counselling, Massage, Reflexology
Details:	All therapies are available to clients and carers on Mondays, Tuesday afternoons, Wednesdays, Thursdays and Friday mornings. Counselling is also open to staff. Self referrals are accepted for all therapies and all require advance booking (clients can be referred by healthcare professional)
Cost:	All free of charge
Quality assurance:	Comprehensive Trust policies on the general use of complementary therapies and on Reflexology
Materials supplied:	Leaflets
Promotion:	Leaflets

Hartlepool and District Hospice

Hilary Sadler   **01429 282100**
13 -15 Hutton Avenue, Hartlepool, Durham TS26 9PW

Therapies:	Aromatherapy, Massage, Relaxation, Visualisation
Details:	All therapies are available to clients on Tuesdays, Thursdays and Fridays, with Aromatherapy and Massage requiring professional referral. Relaxation and Visualisation are available on a drop-in basis
Cost:	All free of charge
Quality assurance:	All patients assessed on first visit and a medical questionnaire is completed. All treatments are given with permission from hospice doctor
Materials supplied:	Information leaflet about Aromatherapy and post-treatment guidelines
Promotion:	All clients are offered service on admission; question on complementary therapies is included on admission documentation; leaflet

Willow Burn Hospice

Margaret Webb   **01207 563103**
Maiden Law Hospital, Lanchester, Durham DH7 0QN

Therapies:	Aromatherapy, Art Therapy, Massage, Music Therapy, Reflexology, Relaxation
Details:	All therapies are available to clients on Wednesday mornings, Thursday mornings and Friday mornings, with Aromatherapy, Massage, Reflexology and Relaxation open to carers and staff. All require professional referral
Cost:	All free of charge
Quality assurance:	Medical consent prior to start of touch therapies. Client admission/assessment prior to treatment
Promotion:	Leaflet; talks to health professionals (eg. district nurse and GP)

Butterwick Hospice & Butterwick House Children's Hospice

Gwyn Featonby, Head of Complementary Therapies **01642 607742**
Middlefield Road, Stockton-on-Tees, Durham TS19 8XN

A specialist palliative care centre, that also incorporates a specialist children's hospice. It offers residential hospice care in Stockton and day care facilities at Stockton and Bishop Auckland

Therapies:	Acupuncture, Aromatherapy, Art Therapy, Counselling, Massage, Meditation, Reflexology, Relaxation, Visualisation
Details:	Practitioners are available Monday to Friday including evenings. Nursing staff with specific complementary therapy skills available 24 hours per day, 7 days per week, offering all therapies to clients, Aromatherapy, Counselling, Massage and Relaxation to carers, and Counselling to staff. Self referrals are accepted for all therapies. All may be advance booked with drop-in available for Aromatherapy, Art Therapy, Massage, Meditation, Reflexology, Relaxation and Visualisation
Cost:	All free of charge
Quality assurance:	Evidence-based policy, protocol and guidelines followed for care. Discussion held in multidisciplinary team meetings prior to treatment commencing. Approval of medical practitioner obtained prior to treating patients. All patients patch tested prior to using essential oils
Materials supplied:	Information leaflets, video and audio tapes used in relaxation
Promotion:	Offered to patients when admitted for day/inpatient/outpatient care; information in hospice booklet; making Macmillan nurses, GPs and hospital units aware of service; leaflets for new patients and carers

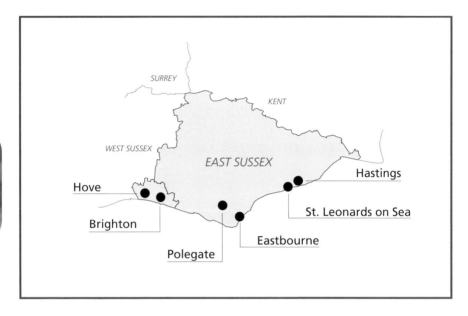

Complementary therapy services in

East Sussex

Brighton	• Royal Sussex County Hospital
Eastbourne	• St Wilfrid's Hospice
Hastings	• Hastings & Rother NHS Trust
Hove	• Macmillan Community Team
	• The Martlets Hospice
Polegate	• Polegate Cancer Support Group
St Leonards on Sea	• Sara Lee Centre

Royal Sussex County Hospital

Hospital Macmillan Team (Colin Twomey)   **01273 664693**
Eastern Road, Brighton, East Sussex BN2 5BE

Therapies:	Aromatherapy, Art Therapy, Counselling, Massage
Details:	All therapies are available to clients with Counselling open to carers. Counselling is available Monday to Friday; Massage and Aromatherapy are available on Friday mornings and Art Therapy is available on Thursday mornings. Self referrals are accepted for all therapies, all must be booked in advance
Cost:	All free of charge
Promotion:	Information leaflets; posters

St Wilfrid's Hospice

Mrs Barbara Cameron, Matron   **01323 644500**
2-4 Mill Gap Road, Eastbourne, East Sussex BN21 2HJ

St Wilfrid's is a specialist palliative care unit that provides inpatient, day and home care, together with bereavement, outpatient, lymphoedema support and educational services

Therapies:	Aromatherapy, Relaxation
Details:	All therapies are available on request to clients, carers and staff on weekdays; all require professional referral
Cost:	All free of charge
Quality assurance:	Aromatherapist is trained. Relaxation provided by a trained complementary therapist and a physiotherapist
Materials supplied:	Relaxation tapes
Promotion:	Clients are advised following a referral to any part of our service

Hastings & Rother NHS Trust

Mrs Gillian Chapple   **01424 755255**
Conquest Hospital, The Ridge, Hastings, East Sussex TN37 7RD

The Trust can be found within the oncology unit of the hospital

Therapies:	Aromatherapy, Massage, Reflexology, Reiki
Details:	All therapies are available to clients and carers on Tuesdays, Wednesdays and Friday mornings. Additionally, Massage is available to staff. Self referrals are accepted
Cost:	Please enquire
Quality assurance:	Assessment by a Macmillan nurse
Promotion:	Leaflets; offered as part of overall treatment

Macmillan Community Team

Lesley Parker   **01273 885000**
The Martlets Hospice, Wayfield Avenue, Hove, East Sussex BN3 7LW

Therapies:	Aromatherapy, Massage, Relaxation, Therapeutic Touch, Visualisation
Details:	All therapies are available to clients and carers on weekdays with Aromatherapy, Massage, Relaxation and Therapeutic Touch available to staff. All therapies must be booked in advance; all require professional referral
Cost:	Please enquire
Materials supplied:	Music Therapy relaxation tapes; Aromatherapy leaflet; information on diet and vitamins
Promotion:	Leaflets distributed to district nurses and GP surgeries; teaching sessions

The Martlets Hospice

Mrs Jenny Musther, Nurse Manager   **01273 273400 x404**
Wayfield Avenue, Hove, East Sussex BN3 7LW

Therapies:	Aromatherapy, Art Therapy, Counselling, Massage, Music Therapy, Relaxation, Nutritional Supplements, Visualisation
Details:	Therapies are available to clients from Monday to Thursday and to staff in the evenings at variable times. Aromatherapy, Counselling and Massage are available to carers and staff. Professional referral is required for all therapies
Cost:	All free of charge
Quality assurance:	Yes for Aromatherapy and Massage
Promotion:	Information brochures for clients and carers

Polegate Cancer Support Group

Miss Pat Harker or Mr Jon Mabey   **01323 485039 or 01424 218355**
24 Walnut Walk, Polegate, East Sussex BN26 5AJ

Therapies:	Meditation, Relaxation, Spiritual Healing, Visualisation
Details:	Therapies are available to clients on Wednesday mornings (10.00–12.00). Self referrals are accepted for all therapies
Cost:	All free of charge
Materials supplied:	Tapes, books and leaflets
Promotion:	Leaflets and posters; through Cancerlink and CancerBACUP; word of mouth

Sara Lee Centre

Mrs Deborah Whitehead, Sara Lee Centre Coordinator   **01424 445177**
St Michael's Hospice, 25 Upper Maze Hill, St Leonards on Sea, East Sussex TN38 0LB

Funded by the Sara Lee Trust, a registered charity, the Sara Lee Centre is situated within St Michael's, an independent, voluntary hospice

Therapies:	Acupuncture, Aromatherapy, Counselling, Massage, Reflexology, Reiki, Relaxation, Shiatsu, Therapeutic Touch, Visualisation
Details:	All therapies except Reiki are available to clients and carers on Mondays, Tuesdays, Wednesday mornings, Thurdays and Fridays, with Reiki available on Tuesday, Thursday and Friday evenings for staff only. On Saturdays, domiciliary visits by appointment. All complementary therapies except Shiatsu are available to staff. While all therapies are available on a drop-in basis, Counselling, Relaxation and Visualisation can be advance booked. Professional referral is required and additionally, staff can self-refer for Reiki
Cost:	Please enquire
Quality assurance:	Assessment is by the Sara Lee Centre co-ordinator. Acupuncture is discussed with the medical team
Materials supplied:	Audiotapes and books are available to loan
Promotion:	Leaflets; information in hospice year book and quarterly newsletters; hospice website; through healthcare professionals who are advised of the Centre's work; through healthcare professionals who attend training/seminars on hospice care

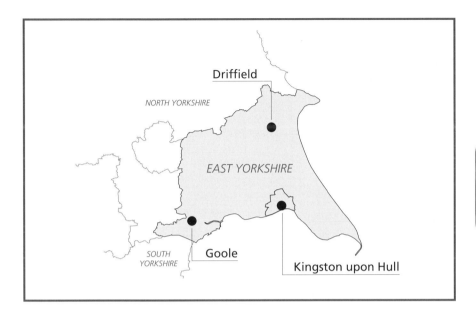

Complementary therapy services in
East Yorkshire

Driffield	● Yorkshire Wolds & Coast PCT NHS Trust
Goole	● Cancer Concern
Kingston upon Hull	● Dove House Hospice

Yorkshire Wolds & Coast PCT NHS Trust

Debbie Simms, Complementary Therapy Sister   **01482 677436**
Alfred Bean Hospital, Bridlington Road, Driffield, East Yorkshire YO25 5JR

The Trust covers three community GP wards, three palliative day care units and a large community/domiciliary caseload

Therapies: Aromatherapy, Massage, Reflexology, Relaxation
Details: All therapies are available on weekdays to clients and carers,
                      with Aromatherapy, Massage and Relaxation also open to
                      staff. All therapies are available on self referral and operate on
                      a drop-in basis
Cost: All free of charge
Quality assurance: Comprehensive referral and assessment forms. Policy,
                      guidelines and protocols in place. Close working relationship
                      with all colleagues enables exchange of information
Materials supplied: Drop-in information groups; leaflet about each therapy;
                      research papers for all to access
Promotion: Leaflets for patients; posters in day care units; letters to GPs,
                      colleagues and ward staff; verbal exchange of information;
                      Cancer Advice Network in East Yorkshire group

Cancer Concern

Margaret Heald   **01757 638050**
9 Downe Close, East Cowick, Goole, East Yorkshire DN14 9EY

Therapies: Aromatherapy, Counselling, Massage, Nutritional Programmes,
                      Relaxation, Spiritual Healing, Nutritional Supplements
Details: Therapies are provided by arrangement at meetings held on
                      the last Thursday of each month and provide the full range of

therapies to carers and staff. Counselling, Nutritional Programmes, Relaxation, Spiritual Healing and Nutritional Supplements are available to clients. Self referrals are accepted but all therapies can be referred by a healthcare professional for Counselling

Cost: All free of charge

Quality assurance: Therapists ensure safety of their therapies

Promotion: Word of mouth; advertising

Dove House Hospice

01482 784343

Chamberlain Road, Kingston upon Hull, East Yorkshire HU8 8DH

Therapies: Aromatherapy, Art Therapy, Counselling, Massage, Music Therapy, Reflexology, Reiki, Relaxation, Nutritional Supplements

Details: All therapies are available on weekdays to clients, with Aromatherapy, Counselling and Massage available to carers and Counselling, Massage and Reflexology available to staff. Art Therapy, Counselling, Music Therapy, Relaxation and Nutritional Supplements are open to self referrals with Aromatherapy, Massage, Reflexology and Reiki requiring professional referral

Cost: All free of charge

Staff are charged for Massage and Reflexology

Quality assurance: Full assessment of patient by qualified practitioner. Liaison with named nurse or multidisciplinary team

Promotion: Included in information and reading material for patients; posters; specific literature

Oncology Health Centres

Mary B Walker, Senior Research Nurse   **01482 676708**

Princess Royal Hospital, Saltshouse Road, Kingston upon Hull

Therapies:	Counselling, Hypnotherapy, Relaxation, Visualisation
Details:	All therapies are available to clients and carers on weekdays through self referral (Hypnotherapy only available to clients)
Cost:	All free of charge
Quality assurance:	All patients are assessed by a behavioural oncology specialist nurse or a clinical psychologist
Materials supplied:	Videotapes
Promotion:	Leaflets distributed to all patients with newly-diagnosed cancer. Radio and television interviews

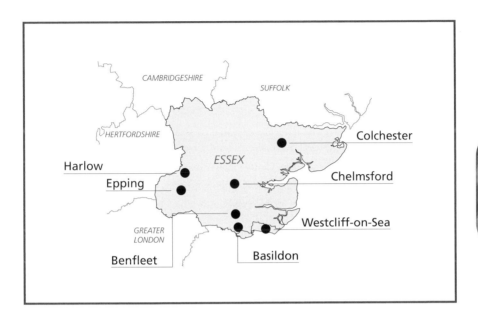

Complementary therapy services in

Essex

Basildon	● St. Luke's Hospice
Benfleet	● Little Haven Children's Hospice
Chelmsford	● Farleigh Hospice
Colchester	● St Helena Hospice
	● The Trinity Centre
Epping	● St Margaret's Hospital
Harlow	● St Clare Hospice
Westcliff-on-Sea	● Fair Havens Hospice

St Luke's Hospice

Jenni Newton, Head of Care Services   **01268 524973**
Fobbing Farm, Nethermayne, Basildon, Essex SS16 5BJ

Therapies:	Aromatherapy, Counselling, Massage, Reflexology, Relaxation
Details:	All therapies are available on weekday mornings (excluding Thursdays) to clients, with Aromatherapy, Counselling, Massage and Reflexology open to carers and staff. Therapies are also available at other times when suitably qualifed staff are available. All therapies require professional referral. Counselling and Relaxation require advance booking (can self-refer for Counselling)
Cost:	All free of charge
Quality assurance:	Require consent from medical practitioner, nurse in charge and patient. Therapists must be qualified and aware of contra-indications
Promotion:	Information folder and in planning care programme; with nurses, for patients and carers; announced at carers support group meeting; announced at staff meetings; word of mouth

Little Haven Children's Hospice

01702 552200
Daws Heath Road, Thundersley, Benfleet, Essex SS7 2LH

Respite care offered for children and their families, and end-of-life care through to bereavement support in a home-from-home setting

Therapies:	Aromatherapy, Art Therapy, Counselling, Herbal Remedies, Homeopathy, Massage, Music Therapy, Nutritional Programmes, Reflexology, Relaxation, Nutritional Supplements, Therapeutic Touch

Details:	Core staff provide services at all times when on shift, making all therapies available to clients most of the week, and Aromatherapy, Art Therapy, Counselling, Massage, Music Therapy, Reflexology and Relaxation available to carers and staff. Self referrals are accepted. Aromatherapy, Massage and Reflexology require advance booking
Cost:	Staff are charged for complementary therapies. Homeopathy and Herbal Remedies are only provided if they are already being used by the client's family
Quality assurance:	Contact with GP/paediatrician and consent from parent before undergoing treatment/therapy
Promotion:	Word of mouth when planning care; leaflets; letters to families

Farleigh Hospice

Ann Smits, Head of Patient Care   **01245 358130**
212 New London Road, Chelmsford, Essex CM2 9AE

Farleigh is a specialist palliative care unit offering inpatient beds, day and community care, and bereavement support; complementary therapies are available to all

Therapies:	Aromatherapy, Art Therapy, Massage, Meditation, Music Therapy, Reiki, Relaxation
Details:	All therapies are available to clients with Aromatherapy, Massage, Meditation, Reiki and Relaxation open to carers and Aromatherapy, Massage, Meditation and Relaxation to staff. Contact for details of availability. Self referrals are accepted but clients can also be referred by healthcare professionals
Cost:	All free of charge
Quality assurance:	Always with consent of patient's clinician. Policy/guidelines available
Promotion:	Word of mouth; hospice leaflets

St Helena Hospice

Ms Ros Christian, Complementary Therapist　　　　　　**01255 221222**
Barncroft Close, Highwoods, Colchester, Essex CO4 4SF

The Hospice offers day, community and inpatient services

Therapies:	Acupuncture, Art Therapy, Counselling, Massage, Shiatsu
Details:	All therapies are available to clients, availability depending on the therapy being offered and the part of the service where the therapy is given. Art Therapy, Counselling, Massage and Shiatsu are available to carers. Professional referrals are required and all therapies must be booked in advance
Cost:	All free of charge
Quality assurance:	All therapists have access to patient records. Each therapist is professionally accountable and takes a history from the patient. Clinical staff are available to discuss with therapist if information is needed
Promotion:	Through referral from any member of the team professionally involved in that person's support

The Trinity Centre

Steve Knowland, Director　　　　　　**01206 561150**
12&21 Trinity Street, Colchester, Essex CO1 1JN

The centre is a registered charity providing a wide range of complementary therapies and activities to improve the health and well being of the whole person

Therapies:	Acupuncture, Aromatherapy, Art Therapy, Chiropractic, Counselling, Herbal Remedies, Homeopathy, Massage, Meditation, Music Therapy, Naturopathy, Osteopathy, Nutritional Programmes, Reflexology, Reiki, Relaxation, Shiatsu, Spiritual Healing, Nutritional Supplements, Visualisation
Details:	Operates a Monday afternoon drop-in healing service; (contact for availability of other therapies). Acupuncture, Aromatherapy,

Art Therapy, Counselling, Herbal Remedies, Homeopathy, Meditation, Music Therapy, Naturopathy, Nutritional Programmes, Reflexology, Reiki, Relaxation, Spiritual Healing, Nutritional Supplements and Visualisation are open to clients and carers. Acupuncture, Aromatherapy, Art Therapy, Chiropractic, Counselling, Herbal Remedies, Homeopathy, Massage, Meditation, Music Therapy, Naturopathy, Osteopathy, Nutritional Programmes, Reflexology, Reiki, Relaxation, Shiatsu, Spiritual Healing, Nutritional Supplements and Visualisation are open to staff. All therapies are open to self referrals and are advance booked except for Spiritual Healing

Cost: Some therapies may be offered free of charge for initial sessions through a bursary fund, which may also reduce fees for further treatments/consultations

Quality assurance: Individual therapists are aware of guidelines on treating cancer patients. Caution is exercised about advising the use of Massage

Materials supplied: Cancer pack about holistic approach includes leaflets, relaxation tape, useful contacts, recommended reading, etc

Promotion: Leaflets; posters; website (www.trinityhealing.org)

St Margaret's Hospital

Judith Spencer-Knoll, Breast Care Specialist Nurse　　　**01279 827301**
Breast Unit, North Weald Road, Epping, Essex CM16 6TN

Therapies: Reflexology
Details: Available on Monday mornings, Tuesdays and Fridays. Professional referral and advance booking are required
Cost: All free of charge
Quality assurance: Health professional directs the therapy as appropriate
Materials supplied: CancerBACUP booklets available; Breast Cancer Care booklets available; in-house Filofax
Promotion: One-to-one advice; collection box for charity that funds the service

St Clare Hospice

Mrs Birgit Gooch   **01279 435431**

Hastingwood Road, Hastingwood, Harlow, Essex CM17 9JX

There is an eight-bed inpatient unit. A day hospice is held at Hastingwood, Saffron Walden and Loughton. Domiciliary visits are also made

Therapies:	Aromatherapy, Counselling, Massage, Reflexology
Details:	All therapies are available to clients from Tuesday to Friday with Counselling also available to carers and staff. Professional referral is required for all therapies, although Counselling may also be self referred; booking is required for Counselling
Cost:	All free of charge
Quality assurance:	Initial assessment made by senior nurse/aromatherapist. Medical permission elicited. Counselling assessment always made by services manager – appointments by arrangement
Promotion:	Word of mouth; information leaflets

Fair Havens Hospice

Catherine Wood, Head of Nursing   **01702 344879**

126 Chalkwell Avenue, Westcliff-on-Sea, Essex SS0 8HN

Therapies:	Aromatherapy, Counselling, Massage
Details:	All therapies are offered to clients and carers, with Counselling and Massage open to staff (there is no fixed availability). Self referrals are accepted for all therapies. Counselling and Massage require advance booking (and clients can be referred by health professional for Counselling)
Cost:	All free of charge
Materials supplied:	CancerBACUP information available
Promotion:	Patient information folder

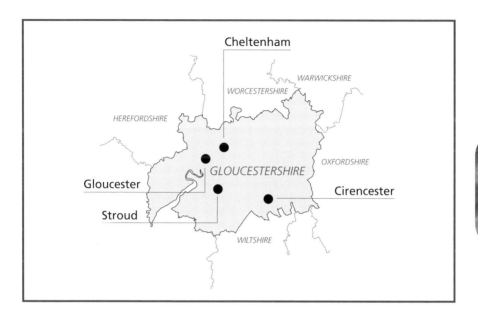

Complementary therapy services in

Gloucestershire

Cheltenham	• Cancer Information Centre
	• East Gloucestershire NHST
Cirencester	• Cirencester Hospital
Gloucester	• Gloucestershire Royal Hospital
	• Wheatstone Day Hospice
Stroud	• Cotswold Care Hospice

Cancer Information Centre

Carol Adams   **01242 274414**

Oncology Unit, Cheltenham General Hospital, Sandford Road, Cheltenham, Gloucestershire GL53 7AN

Therapies:	Counselling, Massage, Reflexology
Details:	Therapies are available to clients on Tuesday afternoons, Wednesday mornings and Friday mornings, with Massage also available to carers. Professional referral is only required for Counselling but all therapies must be booked in advance
Cost:	All free of charge
Promotion:	Posters; leaflets

East Gloucestershire NHST

Sandra Flanagan MHFAF, IIHHT, AOC Registered, BFRP   **01242 273447**
                                                                             01242 679260

Palliative Care Department, Cheltenham General Hospital, Sandford Road, Cheltenham, Gloucestershire GL53 7AN

Therapies:	Aromatherapy, Bach Flower Remedies (or Flower Essences), Massage
Details:	All therapies are available to clients, carers and staff at weekends and every evening. All therapies available on self referral and require advance booking
Cost:	Fees charged for Aromatherapy, Bach Flower Remedies (or Flower Essences), Massage
Quality assurance:	Appropriate and relevant written information is available for every treatment offered. Verbal advice always given before, during and after treatments
Promotion:	Brochure

Cirencester Hospital

Heather Whelan, Personnel Department	**01285 884593**

Tetbury Road, Cirencester, Gloucestershire GL7 1UY

Therapies:	Counselling, Massage, Reflexology
Details:	All therapies available on Mondays, Monday evenings, Thursdays afternoons and evenings for clients, carers and staff. Professional referral required for Counselling only
Cost:	A fee is charged for Massage and Reflexology
Promotion:	Booklet given; staff notices

Gloucestershire Royal Hospital

Dr Alison Duncan	**01452 395179**

Palliative Care Team, Great Western Road, Gloucester, Gloucestershire GL1 3NN

Therapies:	Acupuncture
Details:	Acupuncture is available to clients on weekdays through professional referral. Advance booking is required
Cost:	Please enquire
Quality assurance:	Information given during consultation
Promotion:	Provided as part of clinical service from consultant

Wheatstone Day Hospice

Maria Rainer, Clinical Nurse Manager	**01452 371252**

2 North Upton Lane, Barnwood, Gloucester, Gloucestershire GL4 3TA

This is a day hospice providing specialist palliative care as well as complementary therapies, catering for up to 12 people per day, four days per week

Therapies:	Aromatherapy, Art Therapy, Massage, Reflexology, Reiki, Spiritual Healing

Details:	Therapies are available on weekdays except Tuesdays to clients through self referral
Cost:	All free of charge
Quality assurance:	The patient's GP is asked if they have any objections or if there are any contra-indications. Therapies do not commence until GP has confirmed in writing
Promotion:	Hospice leaflets

Cotswold Care Hospice

Susanne Boyd   **01453 886868**

Longfield, Burleigh Lane, Burleigh, Stroud, Gloucestershire GL5 2PQ

Cotswold Care is a day hospice/hospice-at-home service, providing patient and family support and outpatient complementary therapies

Therapies:	Acupuncture, Aromatherapy, Art Therapy, Massage, Reflexology, Reiki, Relaxation, Nutritional Supplements
Details:	All therapies are available to clients from Monday to Friday, including evenings. Therapies may be used for patients dying at home if appropriate. (Hospice-at-home service operates a 7-days-a-week, 24-hours). Acupuncture, Aromatherapy, Massage, Reflexology and Reiki are available to staff; these therapies plus Art Therapy and Relaxation are also available to carers. Self-referrals are accepted for Aromatherapy, Art Therapy, Massage, Reflexology, Reiki, Relaxation and Nutritional Supplements. Book in advance for Aromatherapy, Art Therapy, Massage, Reflexology, Reiki, Relaxation and Nutritional Supplements
Cost:	All free of charge
Quality assurance:	Consent forms. Policy states assessment and information on side effects for all patients. Review and re-evaluation at regular intervals. Multidisciplinary assessment
Materials supplied:	Information file
Promotion:	Information leaflets; talks; open days; assessment visits

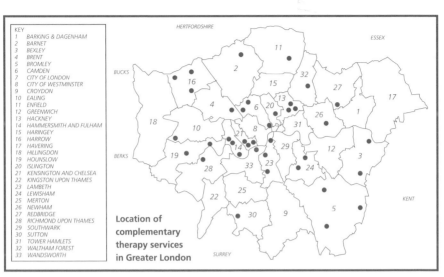

KEY
1 BARKING & DAGENHAM
2 BARNET
3 BEXLEY
4 BRENT
5 BROMLEY
6 CAMDEN
7 CITY OF LONDON
8 CITY OF WESTMINSTER
9 CROYDON
10 EALING
11 ENFIELD
12 GREENWICH
13 HACKNEY
14 HAMMERSMITH AND FULHAM
15 HARINGEY
16 HARROW
17 HAVERING
18 HILLINGDON
19 HOUNSLOW
20 ISLINGTON
21 KENSINGTON AND CHELSEA
22 KINGSTON UPON THAMES
23 LAMBETH
24 LEWISHAM
25 MERTON
26 NEWHAM
27 REDBRIDGE
28 RICHMOND UPON THAMES
29 SOUTHWARK
30 SUTTON
31 TOWER HAMLETS
32 WALTHAM FOREST
33 WANDSWORTH

Location of complementary therapy services in Greater London

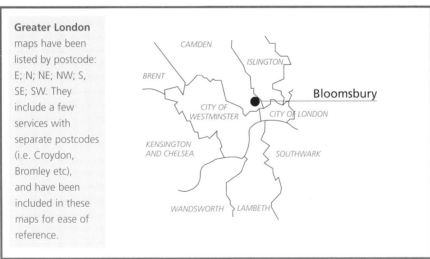

Greater London maps have been listed by postcode: E; N; NE; NW; S, SE; SW. They include a few services with separate postcodes (i.e. Croydon, Bromley etc), and have been included in these maps for ease of reference.

Complementary therapy services in

Central London

Bloomsbury   ● Royal London Homoeopathic Hospital

Royal London Homoeopathic Hospital

Dr Sosie Kassab, Director of Complementary Cancer Services   **020 7837 8833**
Great Ormond Street, Bloomsbury, London WC1N 3HR

Europe's largest public sector service provider of integrated healthcare services, providing complementary treatments for patients with cancer in an outpatient, day care and inpatient setting

Therapies:	Acupuncture, Aromatherapy, Autogenic Training, Homeopathy, Iscador, Massage, Meditation, Reflexology, Reiki, Relaxation, Shiatsu, Visualisation
Details:	Therapies are available to clients on weekdays through professional referral
Cost:	All free of charge
Quality assurance:	All patients are assessed by medical and/or nursing team for appropriateness of individual treatments
Materials supplied:	Leaflets; relaxation tapes
Promotion:	Education to healthcare professionals and patient groups. Leaflets on complementary cancer care programme

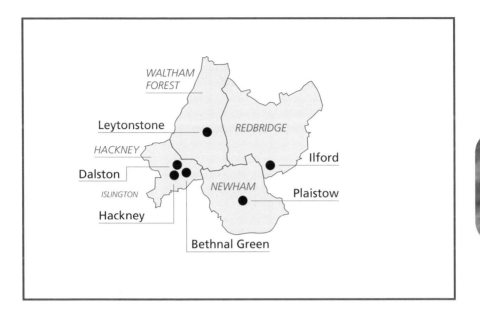

Complementary therapy services in

East London

Bethnal Green	● Mildmay Mission Hospital
Dalston	● Cancer Black Care
Hackney	● St Joseph's Hospice
Ilford	● Barking, Havering & Redbridge Hospitals NHS Trust
Leytonstone	● The Margaret Centre
Plaistow	● Newham Healthcare NHS Trust

Mildmay Mission Hospital

Patricia Waldron   **020 7613 6300**
Hackney Road, Bethnal Green, Greater London E2 7NA

The Mission Hospital is a Christian charity providing services to men, women and children with HIV, AIDS and young physically disabled. It provides rehabilitation, respite, palliative mental health, drug and alcohol care

Therapies:	Aromatherapy, Art Therapy, Massage, Music Therapy, Nutritional Programmes, Relaxation, Nutritional Supplements, Visualisation
Details:	All therapies are available to clients on weekdays, with Massage also available to staff. Self referrals are accepted for Aromatherapy, Art Therapy, Massage, Music Therapy, Relaxation and Visualisation; professional referral is required for Nutritional Programmes, Nutritional Supplements. Drop-in is available for Relaxation
Cost:	Please enquire
Quality assurance:	Through nurse patient assessment. Client focused choice
Materials supplied:	Currently designing leaflets
Promotion:	Newsletter; highlights; conferences; website; word of mouth

Cancer Black Care

Isaac Dweben, Chief Executive   **020 7249 1097**
16 Dalston Lane, Dalston, Greater London E8 3AZ

Therapies:	Aromatherapy, Counselling, Massage, Relaxation, Spiritual Healing
Details:	All therapies are available to clients and carers on Saturday

afternoons through self referral when booked in advance.
Counselling is available on a drop-in basis

Cost: All free of charge

Promotion: By word of mouth and newsletter

St Joseph's Hospice

Maura Cochrane, Assistant Director of Nursing   **020 8525 6000**

Mare Street, Hackney, Greater London E8 4SA

St Joseph's own complementary therapy department, The Wellspring Centre, has
therapy and counselling rooms and a small kitchen for refreshments. Patients give a
very positive response and the centre is always fully booked

Therapies: Acupuncture, Aromatherapy, Art Therapy, Counselling,
Hypnotherapy/Hypnosis, Massage, Meditation, Music Therapy,
Reflexology, Reiki, Relaxation, Shiatsu, Visualisation

Details: All therapies are available to clients, with Acupuncture,
Aromatherapy, Art Therapy, Counselling, Massage,
Reflexology, Reiki, Relaxation, Shiatsu and Visualisation
available to carers, and Aromatherapy, Counselling, Massage,
Reflexology, Reiki, Relaxation, Shiatsu and Visualisation
available to staff. Professional referral required for all therapies
except Aromatherapy, Art Therapy, Meditation, Music Therapy
and Relaxation. Open weekdays for advance bookings only

Cost: All free of charge

Promotion: Leaflets and posters; networking with, eg. hospital palliative
care teams

Barking, Havering & Redbridge Hospitals NHS Trust

Kate Williams, Ward Manager   020 8970 8251
Isobel Donn Day Unit, King George Hospital, Barley Lane, Goodmayes, Ilford, Greater London IG3 8YB

Cancer service day unit

Therapies:	Reflexology
Details:	Reflexology is open to clients on Tuesday afternoons. Both professional and self referrals are accepted. Sessions must be booked in advance
Cost:	All free of charge
Quality assurance:	Information leaflet. Patients can self-refer or be referred by a health professional
Materials supplied:	Leaflets, cassettes, videos
Promotion:	Leaflets; referral through staff

The Margaret Centre

Vivien Hancock or Irene Charter   020 8535 6604
Whipps Cross University Hospital NHS Trust, Whipps Cross Road, Leytonstone, Greater London E11 1NR

The Margaret Centre has a 12-bedded, palliative care unit located in the grounds of Whipps Cross Hospital

Therapies:	Acupuncture, Aromatherapy, Art Therapy, Massage, Reflexology, Relaxation, Shiatsu, Nutritional Supplements, Therapeutic Touch, Visualisation
Details:	All therapies are available to clients on weekdays except Wednesdays, with Massage, Reflexology, Relaxation and Therapeutic Touch open to carers and staff. Professional referral is required for Acupuncture, Aromatherapy, Reflexology and Relaxation. Art Therapy, Massage, Nutritional

	Supplements and Therapeutic Touch are available on self-referral
Cost:	Please enquire
Quality assurance:	Information on side effects, etc. Service is audited. Written information is given
Promotion:	Leaflets; word of mouth
Promotion:	At point of introduction to service for both inpatients and outpatients via leaflets

Newham Healthcare NHS Trust

Clare Darwell   **020 73638105**

Newham General Hospital, Glen Road, Plaistow, Greater London E13 8SL

A district general hospital setting up a small complementary therapy service by autumn 2002

Therapies:	Reflexology
Details:	Reflexology is available to clients via the palliative care team on an advance-booked basis (availability to be planned)
Cost:	All free of charge
Quality assurance:	Will need agreement of oncologist and, if an inpatient, the hospital consultant. Patient's feet and medical history will be assessed by the reflexologist
Promotion:	Poster in the chemotherapy room; leaflets for appropriate outpatient clinics. Appropriate consultants are aware and can refer patients. Palliative care team is providing the service – they also see inpatients

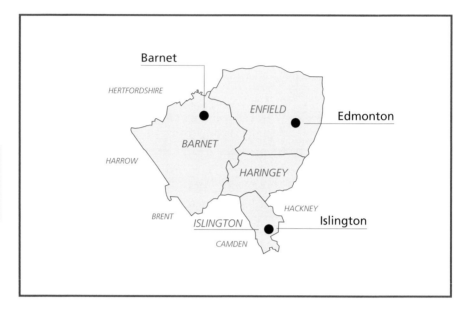

Complementary therapy services in

North London

Barnet	● Cherry Lodge Cancer Care
Edmonton	● North Middlesex University Hospital
Islington	● Cancer Counselling Trust

Cherry Lodge Cancer Care

Mina West, Nurse Service Facilitator **020 8216 4486**

Cherry Lodge, Elmbank, Wood Street, Barnet, Greater London EN5 3HD

Cherry Lodge is an information and resource centre running educational seminars. For complementary therapies it operates an open referral system, drop-in sessions and classes in Chi Kung (Qi Gong) and Yoga. It also provides a befriending service in the community

Therapies:	Acupuncture, Alexander Technique, Aromatherapy, Art Therapy, Counselling, Herbal Remedies, Homeopathy, Massage, Bio-dynamic Massage, Reflexology, Reiki, Relaxation, Spiritual Healing
Details:	All therapies are available to clients and carers from Monday to Thursday with minimal availability on Friday. Also two Thursday evenings a month. Acupuncture, Reiki, Relaxation and Spiritual Healing therapies available to staff as needed and when there is space. All therapies are open to self referrals and drop-ins but all except Reflexology may also be booked. Clients can be referred by healthcare professionals for all therapies
Cost:	All free of charge
Quality assurance:	New members are assessed by a nurse and informed about relevant complementary therapies. Leaflets written by staff are available on most complementary therapies provided
Materials supplied:	Books, Centre-developed leaflets on each complementary therapy
Promotion:	Leaflets, posters, information stalls; fund raising; visits to/from other health professionals who inform clients; members

89

North Middlesex University Hospital

Macmillan Oncology/Palliative Care Team   **020 8887 2475**
Sterling Way, Edmonton, Greater London N18 1QX

Macmillan specialist nurses have provided oncology/palliative care service since 1992, through which complementary therapies were introduced for oncology patients. For five years complementary therapies have been funded by the HEAL Cancer Charity, part of Helen Rollason Cancer Care Centre Appeal

Therapies:	Aromatherapy, Reflexology
Details:	All therapies are available to clients and staff, with Aromatherapy also available to carers. Open on Wednesdays and Thursdays on advance booking only. Self referrals accepted
Cost:	All free of charge
Quality assurance:	Therapies are administered with the prime objective of relaxing the patient. Aromatherapy and Reflexology are considered suitable for most patients. Therapists have training and experience to modify their treatment according to patient's condition
Materials supplied:	Leaflets on how to find an aromatherapist locally; ad hoc reprints of information requested by some patients
Promotion:	Posters

Cancer Counselling Trust

Christine Bradler, Counselling Co-ordinator   **020 7704 1137**
Caspari House, 1 Noel Road, Islington, Greater London N1 8HQ

A counselling service, both face-to-face and by telephone, for anyone affected by cancer, including patients, friends, relatives and those bereaved through cancer

Therapies:	Counselling
Details:	Counselling is available to clients and carers on Monday to Thursday including evenings. All therapies are available on self

referral and must be booked in advance

Cost:	A fee is charged for Counselling
Quality assurance:	Initial telephone assessment; then in-depth assessment with counsellor
Materials supplied:	Leaflets, individual publications when appropriate
Promotion:	Leaflets, posters and website; outreach work with other cancer charities, hospitals, etc

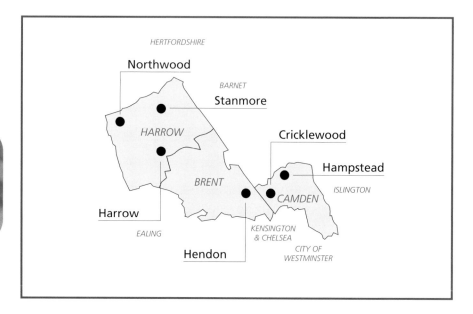

Complementary therapy services in

North West London

Cricklewood	● Natural Death Centre
Hampstead	● Cancerkin
	● Marie Curie Centre - Edenhall
	● Royal Free Hospital
Harrow	● St Luke's Hospice (Harrow & Brent)
Hendon	● Chai Lifeline Cancer Care
Northwood	● Lynda Jackson Macmillan Centre
	● Michael Sobell House
Stanmore	● Royal National Orthopaedic Hospital

Natural Death Centre

Josefine Speyer, Director   **020 8208 2853**

20 Heber Road, Cricklewood, Greater London NW2 6AA

The Centre is an independent, non-profit organisation with two psychotherapists as directors. It aims to support those dying at home and their carers, and to help them arrange funerals

Therapies:	Counselling
Details:	Therapy is available to clients, carers and staff during the day through self referral and by appointment
Cost:	A fee is charged for Counselling
Quality assurance:	Assessment interview
Materials supplied:	We sell the new Natural Death handbook, set of forms including living well and annual journal
Promotion:	'Meetings & Workshops' leaflets states that counselling is available privately with Natural Death Centre directors

Cancerkin

Gloria Freilich or Maureen Hughes   **020 7830 2323**

The Cancerkin Centre, Royal Free Hospital, Pond Street, Hampstead, Greater London NW3 2QG

Although based on the Royal Free site, Cancerkin serves patients and families regardless of where they are treated. It offers complementary therapies, a patient support group, and a Look Good Feel Better programme. The centre and services are being expanded this year

Therapies:	Aromatherapy, Counselling, Yoga
Details:	All therapies are available to clients with Counselling open to carers. Aromatherapy is available all day on Monday and Tuesday to Friday mornings. The Look Good Feel Better

programme and patient group meetings run monthly on Tuesday afternoon and Yoga on Wednesday afternoon. Self referrals are accepted for all therapies. Advance booking is required.

Cost: All free of charge
Volunteer visitors service; Look Good Feel Better service; group support and psychosexual counselling

Quality assurance: Aromatherapy not given until chemotherapy completed; potentially harmful oils excluded. Yoga programme tailored to suit each person's condition. All patients are advised on every aspect of each type of treatment

Promotion: Medical and nursing referrals; leaflets and posters; newsletters; website (www.cancerkin.org.uk); media

Marie Curie Cancer Care – Edenhall

11 Lyndhurst Gardens, Hampstead, Greater London NW3 5NS

Therapies: Acupuncture, Aromatherapy, Art Therapy, Counselling, Hypnotherapy/Hypnosis, Massage, Reflexology, Relaxation, Spiritual Healing, Visualisation

Details: All therapies are open to clients, with Art Therapy, Counselling and Relaxation open to carers, and Counselling, Hypnotherapy/Hypnosis, Reflexology, Relaxation and Spiritual Healing therapies open to staff. Open weekdays and Monday, Tuesday, Thursday and Saturday evenings. Drop-in available for Relaxation; book in advance for: Acupuncture, Aromatherapy, Art Therapy, Counselling, Hypnotherapy/Hypnosis, Massage, Reflexology, Spiritual Healing and Visualisation. Outpatients must be referred by healthcare professionals for Aromatherapy and Massage. Patients may be referred by healthcare

professionals for Art Therapy, Spiritual Healing and
Hypnotherapy/Hypnosis. Clients (usually as inpatients) can self-
refer once they have received a therapy

Cost: All free of charge

Quality assurance: Policies regarding contra-indications. Recommend one touch
therapy at a time. Care packages reviewed in multidisciplinary
team meetings

Promotion: At point of introduction to service for both inpatients and
outpatients via leaflets

Royal Free Hospital

Keith Hunt, Complementary Therapy Co-ordinator   **020 7974 0500 x8927**
Hazzall Ward, Pond Street, Hampstead, Greater London NW3 2QG

The service is for all patients on an inpatient basis who are undergoing cancer
treatment at the Royal Free Hospital

Therapies: Aromatherapy, Massage, Osteopathy, Reflexology

Details: All therapies are available to clients on wards on weekdays
except Wednesday mornings, when they are available in clinic.
Massage and Reflexology are available to staff. Professional
referral and advance booking are required for all therapies

Cost: All free of charge
Fee may apply to staff for Massage & Reflexology

Quality assurance: Doctors referral states what area to be worked on

Materials supplied: Information regarding sleep and relaxation techniques

Promotion: Posters; ward sister; clinic staff

St Luke's Hospice (Harrow & Brent)

Geraldine Burke, Director of Patient Services   **020 8382 8000**

Kenton Grange, Kenton Road, Kenton, Harrow, Greater London HA3 0YG

The Hospice occupies a renovated, listed building. A new build inpatient unit was opened in 2000. As the hospice is in an early stage of development, complementary therapies are limited, but are regarded as a significant component of hospice care, for which further investment is planned

Therapies:	Acupuncture, Aromatherapy, Counselling, Massage, Reflexology, Relaxation
Details:	All therapies are available to clients on weekday mornings and all day Wednesday, with therapists on call on Wednesday and Thursday evenings, and all day Saturday and Sunday. Counselling is also available to carers. Professional referral is required for all therapies
Cost:	All free of charge
Quality assurance:	Patients access complementary therapies through the day care service and the inpatient unit. Please note that all therapists are currently volunteers
Promotion:	Website (www.stlukes-hospice.org)

Chai Lifeline Cancer Care

Barbara Levin, Director of Services   **020 8202 2211**

Shield House, Harmony Way, off Victoria Road, Hendon, Greater London NW4 2BZ

Chai Lifeline is a centre for health and also does outreach work in the community

Therapies:	Aromatherapy, Art Therapy, Counselling, Massage, Meditation, Nutritional Programmes, Reflexology, Reiki, Relaxation, Shiatsu, Spiritual Healing, Nutritional Supplements, Visualisation
Details:	All therapies are available to clients and carers from Monday to Thursday, plus Friday mornings (and Friday afternoons in

summer). Self referrals and advance bookings are accepted for all therapies; though clients can also be referred by a healthcare professional.

Cost: Free or fees charged on a sliding scale/means-tested

Promotion: News media; word of mouth; leaflet distribution; consultants; nurses

Lynda Jackson Macmillan Centre

Cherry Mackie, Complementary Therapy Co-ordinator   **01923 844694**

Mount Vernon Hospital, Rickmansworth Road, Northwood, Greater London   HA6 2RN

Complementary therapies are provided as part of the Centre's cancer support and information service

Therapies: Aromatherapy, Counselling, Massage, Reflexology, Relaxation, Visualisation

Details: All therapies are available to clients on weekdays, with Relaxation and Visualisation also available to carers. All therapies are available through self referral. Counselling, Relaxation and Visualisation are available on a drop-in basis; Aromatherapy, Counselling, Massage and Reflexology should be advance booked (and can be referred by a healthcare professional)

Cost: All free of charge

Quality assurance: Guidelines for use with complementary therapies. Health care advice. Discussion with patient as appropriate

Materials supplied: Patient information series leaflets; videos; books

Promotion: Leaflets; posters; newsletters; mailshot; networks

Michael Sobell House

Kay Eastment   **01923 844302**
Dept. of Palliative Medicine, Mount Vernon Hospital, Rickmansworth Road,
Northwood, Greater London HA6 2RN

Michael Sobell House runs a specialist palliative care unit mainly for people with
cancer. It is situated in the grounds of Mount Vernon Hospital

Therapies:	Aromatherapy, Counselling, Massage, Reflexology, Relaxation, Nutritional Supplements
Details:	All therapies are available to clients on weekdays, with Aromatherapy, Counselling, Massage and Relaxation open to carers, and Aromatherapy and Massage also open to staff. Professional referral is required and drop-in available for Aromatherapy, Counselling, Massage and Relaxation. Complementary therapies are available to patients who have been referred to the palliative care service – patients are not referred just for complementary therapies
Cost:	All free of charge
Quality assurance:	Therapist consults nursing and medical team prior to therapy
Materials supplied:	Relaxation tapes
Promotion:	Leaflets; verbally via Macmillan and community nurses; verbally on referral and on admission

Royal National Orthopaedic Hospital

Julie Woodford, Lead Nurse   **020 8954 2300 bleep 662**
Cancer Services, Brockley Hill, Stanmore, Greater London HA7 4LP

A supra-regional centre for the management of bone and soft tissue sarcomas and
complex skeletal malignancy

Therapies:	Counselling, Relaxation, Visualisation

Details: All therapies are available to clients and carers on Monday to Saturday mornings. Self referrals accepted for all therapies (can be referred by healthcare professional)

Cost: All free of charge

Materials supplied: CancerBACUP information booklet

Promotion: Referral from professionals in the service

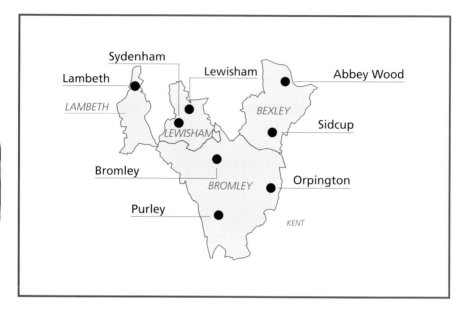

Complementary therapy services in

South East London

Abbey Wood	● Greenwich & Bexley Cottage Hospice
Bromley	● ABACUS Cancer Self Help & Support Group
Lambeth	● Richard Dimbleby Cancer Information & Support Service
Lewisham	● University Hospital Lewisham
Orpington	● Bromley Hospitals NHS Trust
Purley	● South East Cancer Help Centre
Sidcup	● CAMEO Support Group
	● The Douglas Macmillan Cancer Information Centre
Sydenham	● St Christopher's Hospice

Greenwich & Bexley Cottage Hospice

Caroline Ellis, Day Hospice Nurse Manager   **020 8312 2244**
185 Bostall Hill, Abbey Wood, Greater London SE2 0GB

Therapies: Aromatherapy, Counselling, Massage, Meditation, Reflexology, Reiki, Relaxation, Shiatsu, Spiritual Healing, Nutritional Supplements, Visualisation

Details: All therapies are available to clients on weekdays, with Aromatherapy, Counselling, Massage, Meditation, Reflexology, Reiki, Relaxation, Spiritual Healing and Visualisation available to carers and staff; Shiatsu is also available to staff. Both booked and drop-in sessions are available for Aromatherapy, Counselling, Massage, Meditation, Reflexology, Reiki, Relaxation, Shiatsu, Spiritual Healing and Visualisation. Professional referral is required

Cost: All free of charge to clients and carers if booked in advance. Payment from staff for complementary therapies. Payment from patients and carers for complementary therapies provided by drop-in service

Quality assurance: Guidelines; consent from doctor or nurse manager. Access to patients' medical notes. Disclaimers for drop-in service

Materials supplied: Leaflets

Promotion: Leaflets; posters; information packs

ABACUS Cancer Self Help & Support Group

Ray Bailey or Jean Collings   **am/pm: 020 8467 2565 or pm: 020 8325 9546**
16 Southwood Close, Bromley, Greater London BR1 2LU

The ABACUS help line (020 8467 2565) provides support and information to those who make their first contact or who do not wish to attend group meetings. These meetings offer mutual support to people with cancer and their carers. Refreshments are provided

Therapies: Aromatherapy, Massage, Meditation, Nutritional Programmes,

	Reflexology, Relaxation, Spiritual Healing, Visualisation
Details:	All therapies are available to clients, carers and staff on weekdays (weekday evenings by special arrangement). Self referrals are accepted for all therapies. Advance booking is required for Aromatherapy, Massage, Nutritional Programmes, Reflexology and Spiritual Healing therapies; drop-in available for Meditation, Relaxation, Spiritual Healing and Visualisation
Cost:	Free of charge for Meditation, Nutritional Programmes, Relaxation, Spiritual Healing, Visualisation. Fees for Aromatherapy, Massage, Reflexology
Quality assurance:	Therapist is fully qualified and has undertaken additional training to enable her to work with cancer patients (e.g. at Bristol Cancer Help Centre, Marie Curie Cancer Care, Penarth, etc.). Also received advanced training in Aromatherapy and Aromachemistry
Materials supplied:	Tapes to help people relax at home and a variety of helpful books
Promotion:	Complementary therapy service is described in information pack, which also includes nutritional information

Richard Dimbleby Cancer Information & Support Service

Karen Loxton, Complementary Therapy Co-ordinator   **020 7960 5689**
2nd Floor Lambeth Wing, St Thomas' Hospital, Lambeth Palace Road, Lambeth, Greater London SE1 7EH

The Service forms part of a cancer information and support network within a hospital setting, with funding for complementary therapies provided by the Richard Dimbleby Cancer Fund

Therapies:	Aromatherapy, Art Therapy, Counselling, Reflexology, Relaxation, Visualisation
Details:	Therapies are available to clients on weekdays except Tuesday.

Self referrals are accepted for all therapies; Relaxation can be provided on drop-in, but all other therapies should be booked

Cost: All free of charge

Quality assurance: Procedures are outlined in the unit's complementary therapy operational policy. Liaison with healthcare professionals involved in patient's care when necessary

Materials supplied: Leaflets and hand-outs about therapies, how to find a therapist, home use of Aromatherapy oils

Promotion: Leaflets; posters

University Hospital Lewisham

Macmillan Palliative Care Team, Lewisham High Street, Lewisham, Greater London SE13 6LH

Therapies: Counselling, Massage, Reflexology, Relaxation, Visualisation

Details: All therapies are available to clients and carers on Friday mornings, with Counselling, Reflexology, Relaxation and Visualisation also available to staff. All therapies require professional referral and advance booking

Cost: Free of charge for Counselling, Relaxation, Visualisation There is a fee for Reflexology

Quality assurance: Trained, experienced staff assess patients' situations and treat accordingly

Promotion: Team tells patients about the service

Bromley Hospitals NHS Trust

Dee Bryan, Aromatherapist   **01689 814096**

Chartwell Unit, Farnborough Hospital, Farnborough Common, Orpington, Greater London BR6 8ND

The Chartwell Cancer Unit provides an outpatient service for patients with one of the common cancers. Specialist multidisciplinary teams include specialist nurses, doctors, a counsellor and an aromatherapist

Therapies:	Aromatherapy, Counselling, Massage, Nutritional Supplements
Details:	All therapies are available to clients on Fridays, with Aromatherapy, Counselling and Massage also available to carers. All therapies require professional referral and advance booking
Cost:	All free of charge
Quality assurance:	Protocol approved by Trust's board includes: referral criteria; referral form including details of patient's condition; guidance on the use of oils and therapies for individual patients
Materials supplied:	Locally and nationally developed literature
Promotion:	Leaflets; posters; staff recommend the service and refer patients

South East Cancer Help Centre

Kathleen Behan, Co-ordinator   **020 8668 0974**
2 Purley Road (Tesco Development), Purley, Greater London CR8 2HA

Therapies:	Aromatherapy, Art Therapy, Counselling, Drama Therapy, Meditation, Reflexology, Reiki, Relaxation, Shiatsu, Spiritual Healing, Visualisation
Details:	All therapies are available to clients and carers on weekdays and Tuesday, Wednesday, Thursday and Friday evenings. Book in advance for Aromatherapy, Counselling, Meditation, Reflexology, Reiki, Relaxation, Shiatsu, Spiritual Healing and Visualisation; Art Therapy and Drama Therapy are available on drop-in. Self referral accepted for all therapies
Cost:	All free of charge
Quality assurance:	Permission is sought from consultant before giving Aromatherapy, Reflexology and Shiatsu
Materials supplied:	Information pack containing details of all the therapies offered
Promotion:	Leaflets; posters; information packages

CAMEO Support Group

Ted Alger   **020 8303 1487**

The Douglas Macmillan Cancer Information Centre, Queen Mary's Hospital, Frognal
Avenue, Sidcup, Greater London DA14 6LT

The Group meets on the first Wednesday of every month at the Douglas Macmillan
Cancer Information Centre at Queen Mary's Hospital, Sidcup

Therapies:	Aromatherapy, Counselling, Reflexology, Relaxation, Spiritual Healing, Visualisation
Details:	All therapies are available to clients, with Counselling, Relaxation, Spiritual Healing and Visualisation open to carers on the first Wednesday of each month (10.30–12.00). Book in advance for Aromatherapy, Counselling and Reflexology; drop-in available for Spiritual Healing and clients can be referred by healthcare professional for Aromatherapy and Reflexology. Self referrals accepted on all therapies
Cost:	All free of charge
Materials supplied:	Videos and leaflets; fully equipped library on site
Promotion:	Goldshield brochures available at meetings; posters in hospital

The Douglas Macmillan Cancer Information Centre

Manager   **020 8308 3295**

Queen Mary's Hospital, Frognal Avenue, Sidcup, Greater London DA14 6LT

Therapies:	Aromatherapy, Reflexology, Relaxation
Details:	All therapies are available to clients and carers on Tuesday mornings, Thursdays and Friday afternoons, to be booked in advance. Professional referral is required for Aromatherapy and Reflexology

Cost:	All free of charge
Quality assurance:	All therapists are accredited and advise patients of any possible side effects
Promotion:	Leaflets and posters distributed throughout the hospital, GP surgeries and community

St Christopher's Hospice

Liz Hawkins, CT Co-ordinator   **020 8768 4611/4500**

51-59 Lawrie Park Road, Sydenham, Greater London SE26 6DZ

Therapies:	Acupuncture, Aromatherapy, Art Therapy, Counselling, Massage, Reflexology, Relaxation
Details:	All therapies are available to clients Monday to Thursday and Friday mornings, with Aromatherapy, Counselling, Massage and Reflexology also open to carers. Therapies are also available to carers on Sunday mornings. Self referrals are accepted for all therapies and clients can also be referred by health professionals. Book in advance for Acupuncture, Aromatherapy, Counselling, Massage, Reflexology and Relaxation
Cost:	All free of charge
Promotion:	Leaflets

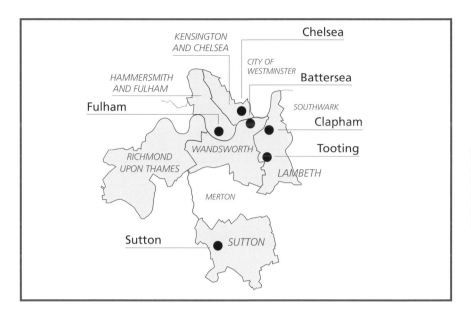

Complementary therapy services in

South West London

Battersea	• The Cancer Resource Centre
Chelsea	• The Royal Marsden NHS Trust
Clapham	• Trinity Hospice
Fulham	• Chelsea and Westminster NHS Trust
	• The Haven Trust
Sutton	• Healing Friends
Tooting	• St George's Healthcare NHS Trust

The Cancer Resource Centre

020 7924 3924

20-22 York Road, Battersea, Greater London SW11 3QE

The Cancer Resource Centre is a voluntary organisation in a community setting

Therapies:	Aromatherapy, Art Therapy, Counselling, Massage, Meditation, Reflexology, Reiki, Relaxation, Shiatsu, Spiritual Healing, Visualisation
Details:	Relaxation and Visualisation therapies are available Monday afternoons; Massage on Tuesday afternoons and Wednesday mornings, Counselling on Thursday afternoons, Meditation on Friday afternoons. Times vary for other therapies. All therapies are available to clients with all except Shiatsu open to carers, and Aromatherapy, Counselling, Massage, Meditation, Reflexology, Reiki, Relaxation, Spiritual Healing and Visualisation open to staff. (Shiatsu is only available during home visits). Self referrals accepted for all therapies except Shiatsu
Cost:	Please enquire
Quality assurance:	Initial interviews/assessments are conducted before offering one-to-one therapies. Consent is sought by client from main medical practitioner before any form of Massage is offered. Therapies may be limited; for example, no visualisation/group work for mentally unstable/psychiatric problems
Materials supplied:	Introductory leaflet; lending library of books and tapes
Promotion:	Leaflets and posters in health settings; links with health professionals; articles in papers and magazines

The Royal Marsden NHS Trust

Anne McLean, Rehabilitation Secretary   **020 7808 2811**
Fulham Road, Chelsea, Greater London SW3 6JJ

The Royal Marsden provides complementary therapies for inpatients and outpatients under the Trust's medical care. The Trust is on two sites, Chelsea and Sutton

Therapies:	Acupuncture, Aromatherapy, Art Therapy, Counselling, Massage, Nutritional Programmes, Reflexology, Relaxation, Spiritual Healing, Nutritional Supplements, Visualisation
Details:	Therapies are available on weekdays. For clients: Acupuncture, Aromatherapy, Art Therapy, Counselling, Massage, Nutritional Programmes, Relaxation, Spiritual Healing, Nutritional Supplements and Visualisation. For carers: Aromatherapy, Art Therapy, Counselling, Massage, Relaxation and Visualisation. For staff: Counselling and Reflexology. Professional referral is required for Acupuncture. Aromatherapy, Art Therapy, Counselling, Massage, Nutritional Programmes, Relaxation, Spiritual Healing, Nutritional Supplements and Visualisation available on self referral. Book in advance for Acupuncture, Aromatherapy, Art Therapy, Counselling, Massage, Nutritional Programmes, Relaxation, Spiritual Healing, Nutritional Supplements and Visualisation. (Can be referred by healthcare professional)
Cost:	Fee for staff or private patients
Quality assurance:	This information is provided by the therapist offering the treatment
Materials supplied:	Rehabilitation services leaflet
Promotion:	Leaflets

Trinity Hospice

Jan Wilkinson, Complementary Therapy Co-ordinator   **020 7787 1000**
30 Clapham Common North Side, Clapham, Greater London SW4 0RN

Therapies:	Aromatherapy, Art Therapy, Massage, Reflexology, Relaxation
Details:	All therapies are available to clients; Aromatherapy and Massage available to carers and staff; additionally Reflexology is available to staff. Open weekday mornings (09.30-13.00) and one Saturday per month for inpatients only; Wednesday evenings (17.30-19.30) for carers only and Thursday evenings (17.00-19.00) for staff only. Self-referrals are accepted for Relaxation, Aromatherapy, Massage, Reflexology and Art Therapy for day care and inpatients. Referral by healthcare professionals for Relaxation, Aromatherapy and Massage for community patients. Book in advance for Relaxation, Aromatherapy and Massage for outpatients and carers
Cost:	All free of charge
	There is a fee for therapies for staff
Quality assurance:	Therapist training. Policies. Guidelines and protocols of practice
Materials supplied:	Leaflets, CD for relaxation
Promotion:	Leaflets; via the multiprofessional team

Chelsea and Westminster NHS Trust

Macmillan Support Team   **020 8746 8499**
Chelsea and Westminster Hospital, 369 Fulham Road, Fulham, Greater London SW10 9NH

Therapies:	Counselling
Available:	Counselling is available to clients, carers and staff for half a

day per week to suit patient needs. Professional referral and
advance booking are required

Cost: All free of charge
Fee will apply for staff

Quality assurance: Psychologist must receive written referral stating issues

Promotion: Inform patient if felt appropriate by clinician

The Haven Trust

Louise Webster Goodwin **08707 272273**
Effie Road, Fulham, Greater London SW6 1TB

The Haven Trust is a registered charity, entirely self-funded by donations and grants
from trusts and foundations. All services are provided free of charge

Therapies: Acupuncture, Alexander Technique, Aromatherapy, Art
Therapy, Counselling, Herbal Remedies, Homeopathy,
Massage, Meditation, Nutritional Programmes, Reflexology,
Reiki, Relaxation, Shiatsu, Spiritual Healing, Nutritional
Supplements, Therapeutic Touch, Visualisation

Details: Open weekdays. All therapies are available to clients, and all
except Nutritional Supplements are available to carers. Self
referrals are accepted for all therapies. Advance booking is
required for all therapies except Spiritual Healing

Cost: Free of charge for Acupuncture, Alexander Technique,
Aromatherapy, Art Therapy, Counselling, Herbal Remedies,
Homeopathy, Massage, Meditation, Nutritional Programmes,
Reflexology, Reiki, Relaxation, Shiatsu, Spiritual Healing,
Therapeutic Touch andVisualisation
There is a fee for Supplements

Quality assurance:	To access any treatment, a client must make an appointment with a breast care nurse who will take down a full medical history. Then an individualised plan of treatment is devised. Regular follow-ups with the breast care nurse are planned and treatments altered if necessary
Materials supplied:	Wide range of literature, videos and tapes, including the Bristol Cancer Help Centre's video
Promotion:	Leaflets sent to hospitals and clinics in Greater London; via media articles; via website (www.thehaventrust.org.uk) and links from other sites; word of mouth from current visitors; via open evenings at the centre for breast care nurses and other healthcare professionals

Healing Friends

Marilyn Smith or Glynis Catton   **01737 249950 or 020 8644 2042**

The Friends Meeting House, Cedar Road, Sutton SM2

Healing Friends is a caring group of friends who support each other; with the hand of friendship, they offer kindness, compassion and healing

Therapies:	Art Therapy, Cranio-Sacral Therapy, Meditation, Reflexology, Relaxation, Spiritual Healing, Therapeutic Touch, Visualisation
Details:	All therapies are available on Monday evenings to clients, carers and staff. Self referrals are accepted for all therapies. Book in advance for Art Therapy, Meditation, Reflexology, Relaxation, Spiritual Healing, Therapeutic Touch and Visualisation; drop in for Meditation, Reflexology, Relaxation, Spiritual Healing, Therapeutic Touch and Visualisation
Cost:	A fee is charged for Art Therapy, Cranio-Sacral Therapy, Meditation, Reflexology, Relaxation, Spiritual Healing, Therapeutic Touch and Visualisation
Promotion:	Advertisements

St George's Healthcare NHS Trust

Tina Glynn, Senior Nurse, Palliative Care   **020 8725 3311**

Palliative Care Team, Claire House, St George's Hospital, Blackshaw Road, Tooting, Greater London SW17 0QT

A small service currently covers patients who are referred to the oncology ward and the chemotherapy day unit

Therapies:	Aromatherapy, Counselling, Massage, Reflexology
Details:	All therapies are available to clients, carers and staff on Wednesday and Thursday mornings. Professional referral and advance booking are required for all therapies
Cost:	All free of charge
Quality assurance:	Therapists follow guidelines which outline contra-indications to therapies
Promotion:	Posters; client booklet contains section about complementary therapy service; staff promotion

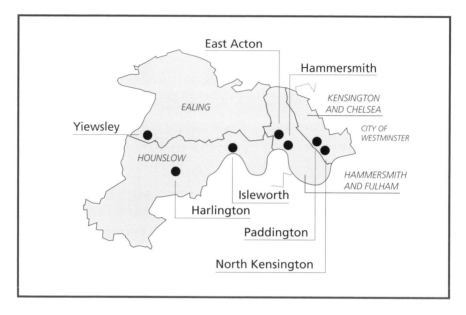

East Acton

Hammersmith

KENSINGTON
AND CHELSEA

EALING

Yiewsley

CITY OF
WESTMINSTER

HOUNSLOW

HAMMERSMITH
AND FULHAM

Isleworth

Harlington

Paddington

North Kensington

Complementary therapy services in

West London

East Acton	• Hammersmith Hospitals NHS Trust (Hammersmith)
Hammersmith	• Hammersmith Hospitals NHS Trust (Charing Cross)
Harlington	• Harlington Hospice
Isleworth	• The Mulberry Centre
North Kensington	• The Pembridge Palliative Care Centre
Paddington	• St. Mary's Hospital
Yiewsley	• Community Cancer Support Centre

Hammersmith Hospitals NHS Trust (Hammersmith Hospital)

Lucy Bell, Complementary Therapy Team Leader   **020 8383 0463**

Hammersmith Hospital, Du Cane Road, East Acton, Greater London W12 0HS

Complementary therapy is an integral part of a multidisciplinary approach to specialist cancer and palliative care. The service is provided to inpatients and outpatients receiving treatment for cancer at both Charing Cross and Hammersmith Hospitals

Therapies:	Aromatherapy, Art Therapy, Counselling, Massage, Reflexology, Relaxation, Visualisation
Details:	All therapies are available to clients, with Counselling, Relaxation and Visualisation available to carers, and Counselling and Massage available to staff. Open on weekdays; self referrals and professional referrals accepted for all therapies. Aromatherapy, Art Therapy, Counselling, Massage and Reflexology require advance booking; drop-in groups for Art Therapy, Relaxation and Visualisation
Cost:	All free of charge
Quality assurance:	Referral forms and guidelines for staff referring patients; doctor to give permission for therapy. Letters sent to consultants notifying them of therapies that their patients are receiving. Policy for use of complementary therapies
Materials supplied:	All patients receive a complementary therapy leaflet: possible benefits, how complementary therapies are used, which ones are on offer and how to access them. List of linked centres in the community and where complementary therapies can be accessed once hospital treatment has finished; lending library of books/tapes
Promotion:	Information leaflets; posters; word of mouth; medical and nursing staff inform patients

Hammersmith Hospitals NHS Trust (Charing Cross Hospital)

Lucy Bell, Complementary Therapy Team Leader   **020 8383 0463**

Charing Cross Hospital, Fulham Palace Road, Hammersmith, Greater London W6 8RF

The complementary therapy service is an integral part of a multidisciplinary approach to specialist cancer and palliative care. The service is provided to inpatients and outpatients receiving treatment for cancer at both Charing Cross and Hammersmith Hospitals

Therapies:	Aromatherapy, Art Therapy, Counselling, Massage, Reflexology, Relaxation, Visualisation
Details:	All therapies are available to clients, with Counselling, Relaxation and Visualisation available to carers, and Counselling and Massage available to staff. Open on weekdays; self referrals accepted for all therapies. Aromatherapy, Art Therapy, Counselling, Massage and Reflexology require advance booking; drop-in service available for Art Therapy, Relaxation and Visualisation; drop-in groups for Relaxation and Visualisation
Cost:	All free of charge
Quality assurance:	Referral form and guidelines for staff referring patients. Doctor to give permission and letter sent to patient's consultant notifying them of complementary therapy being given. Policy for use of complementary therapies. Guidelines and procedures for therapists, including contra-indications
Materials supplied:	Library of books and tapes which can be borrowed; information leaflet which explains: how complementary therapies are used, how patients may benefit and where they can access complementary therapies in the community once they have finished their treatment at the Trust
Promotion:	Information leaflets; posters; word of mouth; medical and nursing staff inform patients

Harlington Hospice

Michele Hodkinson, Care Services Manager   **020 8759 0453**
St Peter's Way, Harlington, Greater London UB3 5AB

Harlington is a day hospice

Therapies:	Aromatherapy, Massage, Reflexology, Reiki, Relaxation
Details:	Open to clients for all therapies on Monday to Thursday mornings. Self referrals are accepted for all therapies
Cost:	All free of charge
Promotion:	Users of the day hospice; via referral agents

The Mulberry Centre

Rita Wilson   **020 8321 6300**
West Middlesex University Hospital, Twickenham Road, Isleworth, Greater London TW7 6AF

The Mulberry Centre is a new walk-in cancer support centre within the grounds of West Middlesex University Hospital, but it is funded entirely by charitable donations. The centre offers support and information to cancer patients of all ages, their families, carers and friends

Therapies:	Aromatherapy, Massage, Meditation, Reflexology, Relaxation, Visualisation
Details:	All therapies are available to clients and carers through self referral. Therapies are available on weekdays, alternate Thursday evenings and one Saturday morning per month. All must be booked in advance. T'ai Chi and Yoga are being introduced this year
Cost:	All free of charge
Quality assurance:	Medical history obtained. Note sent to GP/consultant, but only

with visitor's approval/consent. Therapists receive cancer-specific training to alert them to contra-indications, etc

Materials supplied: Leaflet and access to information library

Promotion: Posters; leaflets; local press; hospitals and GP/nurse specialists; listings in directories

The Pembridge Palliative Care Centre

Dr Anne Naysmith **020 8962 4406**

Parkside Health NHS Trust, St Charles' Hospital, Exmoor Street, North Kensington, Greater London W10 6DZ

The Care Centre is an NHS-funded, specialist palliative care unit, with inpatient and day care facilities. It also has a specialist palliative care community team

Therapies: Aromatherapy, Art Therapy, Massage, Reflexology, Relaxation, Nutritional Supplements

Details: All therapies are available to clients on weekdays and Sunday mornings, with Aromatherapy, Massage and Reflexology also available to staff. Professional referral is required for Aromatherapy, Massage, Reflexology and Nutritional Supplements. Art Therapy and Relaxation are available on self-referral

Cost: All free of charge

Materials supplied: Information on resources available in the locality

Promotion: Information leaflets; information folders; posters

St Mary's Hospital

Joan McCoy, Clinical Nurse Specialist Oncology   **020 7886 6080**

Oncology Department, 4th Floor, Clarence Wing, Praed Street, Paddington, Greater London W2 1NY

Therapies:	Aromatherapy, Counselling, Massage, Reflexology
Details:	All therapies are available to clients Monday to Thursday mornings, with Counselling also open to carers. Professional referral is required for Aromatherapy, Massage and Reflexology; advance booking is necessary for all therapies. Relaxation classes are to be arranged if space can be found
Cost:	All free of charge
Quality assurance:	Referral form for therapies completed by health professional outlining diagnosis, surgery, current and planned treatments
Promotion:	Advertised in chemotherapy department; advertised in patient information leaflets; patients informed through specialist nurses, eg. breast cancer, palliative care, lung cancer, etc

Community Cancer Support Centre

Cherry Mackie, Centre Co-ordinator   **01895 461016**

18a Fairfield Road, Yiewsley, Greater London UB7 8EX

Opened in 1999 just off Yiewsley High Street with volunteers, the centre now has two paid workers. It provides support and information for people affected by cancer

Therapies:	Aromatherapy, Massage, Reflexology, Relaxation, Visualisation
Details:	All therapies are available to clients, carers and staff on weekdays, Wednesday evenings and Saturday mornings. Self referrals and advance bookings are accepted for all therapies
Cost:	Please enquire

Quality assurance: Guidelines and policies adopted from the Lynda Jackson Macmillan Centre. Therapists always takes patient's full history. Records are kept. A discussion always takes place before a patient comes for treatment

Materials supplied: Own in-house leaflets, videos and books

Promotion: Leaflets and posters in hospitals, GPs' surgeries and libraries; networking with local organisations; advertising through shop window; newsletter

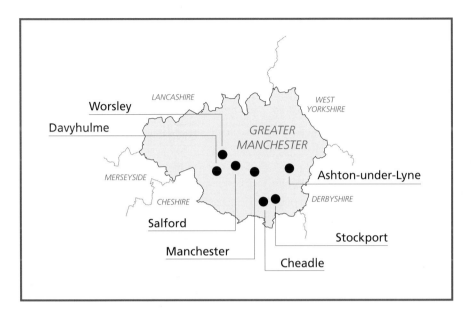

Complementary therapy services in

Greater Manchester

Ashton-under-Lyne	• Willow Wood Hospice
Cheadle	• St Ann's Hospice
Davyhulme	• Trafford Macmillan Care Centre
Manchester	• Christie Hospital NHS Trust
	• Neil Cliffe Cancer Care Centre
Salford	• BASIC (Brain & Spinal Injury Charity)
Stockport	• Beechwood Cancer Care Centre
Worsley	• St Ann's Hospice

Willow Wood Hospice

Barbara Robinson, Matron   **0161 330 1100**

Willow Wood Close, Mellor Road, Ashton-under-Lyne, Greater Manchester OL6 6SL

Therapies:	Acupuncture, Aromatherapy, Art Therapy, Massage, Meditation, Music Therapy, Reflexology, Reiki, Relaxation, Shiatsu, Spiritual Healing
Details:	All therapies are available to clients Monday to Thursday with Acupuncture, Aromatherapy, Massage, Meditation, Reflexology, Reiki, Relaxation, Shiatsu and Spiritual Healing also available to staff. Professional referral is necessary for Acupuncture, Aromatherapy, Art Therapy, Massage, Music Therapy, Reflexology, Reiki, Shiatsu and Spiritual Healing; self referrals are accepted for Meditation and Relaxation
Cost:	All free of charge
Quality assurance:	Policy in place
Materials supplied:	Information folder
Promotion:	Mentioned in general information and day hospice leaflets

St Ann's Hospice

Ann Carter, Complementary Therapy Co-ordinator   **0161 291 2912**

St Ann's Road North, Heald Green, Cheadle, Greater Manchester SK8 3SZ

Therapies:	Aromatherapy, Reflexology, Reiki
Details:	All therapies are available to inpatients Monday to Friday afternoons; to day care outpatients on weekdays except Tuesdays. Therapies may be offered in the evenings by nurse therapists if available on night shift. Clients can self-refer for therapies where a treatment programme is devised by a healthcare professional

Cost: All free of charge

Materials supplied: Information about complementary therapies by everyone's bedside; outpatient day care service supported by information leaflets

Promotion: Service supported by specially written leaflets; through referral from healthcare professionals

Trafford Macmillan Care Centre

Jill Bailey, Head of Complementary Therapy Service   **0161 746 2080**

Trafford General Hospital, Moorside Road, Davyhulme, Greater Manchester M41 5SN

The Care Centre is a cancer information and support centre providing day therapy

Therapies: Acupuncture, Aromatherapy, Art Therapy, Counselling, Massage, Nutritional Programmes, Reflexology, Relaxation, Shiatsu, Nutritional Supplements, Visualisation

Details: All therapies are available to clients and carers on Mondays, Tuesday afternoons, Wednesdays, Thursday afternoons and Friday afternoons. The Centre is planning a complementary therapy service from February 2002 (17.00 – 19.00 Monday to Thursday). Aromatherapy, Massage, Reflexology and Shiatsu are also open to staff. Both self and professional referrals are accepted for all therapies (clients self-refer to the centre in the first instance and then must be referred on by a healthcare professional). Advance booking is required

Cost: Free of charge to clients and carers. A charge is made for staff

Quality assurance: All clients/carers assessed by keyworker – health professional with training in contra-indications. Centre's complementary therapy policy includes referral details and contra-indications for each complementary therapy. Each client/carer assessed by complementary therapy therapist. Head of complementary therapy service monitors compliance with above procedures

Materials supplied:	Leaflets and books on complementary therapies available; website from 2002
Promotion:	Leaflets on the centre and its specialist services; keyworker assessment; client users' group 2002; talks to user groups and health professionals; website and local cancer services directory being developed in 2002

Christie Hospital NHS Trust

Peter A Mackereth, Complementary Therapy Practitioner & Lecturer   0161 446 3795

Wilmslow Road, Withington, Manchester, Greater Manchester M20 4BX

The Christie Hospital is a specialist hospital mainly concerned with treating cancer and associated diseases. It is the largest treatment centre in Europe with over 10,000 new patients registering annually for treatments such as radiotherapy, chemotherapy and surgery

Therapies:	Acupuncture, Aromatherapy, Art Therapy, Counselling, Massage, Chair Massage, Reflexology, Relaxation, Therapeutic Touch, Visualisation
Details:	All therapies are available to clients on a first-come, first-served basis, or a series of booked sessions (contact for details of availability). Counselling, Massage, Chair Massage, Reflexology, Relaxation, Therapeutic Touch and Visualisation are available to carers, and Counselling and Chair Massage to staff. Self referrals are accepted for all therapies and can also be referred by healthcare professional. Advance booking is required for therapies except Aromatherapy and Chair Massage
Cost:	Free to clients and carers; charges apply for staff
Quality assurance:	Policy documents available on all wards/departments – criteria for referral. Referral forms ask for specific information. Complementary therapy practitioner is contacted to discuss

options/understanding/identification and contracting for
appropriate intervention

Materials supplied: Currently literature only; developing intranet site; short video
being considered

Promotion: Leaflets in all clinical areas; posters; newsletters and talks to staff
who make referrals; Manchester-wide palliative care/comple-
mentary therapy meetings; patients inform other patients. There
is a cancer information officer

Neil Cliffe Cancer Care Centre

Ann Carter, Complementary Therapy Co-ordinator   **0161 291 2912**

St Ann's Hospice, Wythenshawe Hospital, Southmoor Road, Manchester, Greater
Manchester M23 9LT

The Care Centre is based at Wythenshawe Hospital but serves the whole community

Therapies: Acupuncture, Aromatherapy, Counselling, Cranio-Sacral
Therapy, Homeopathy, Massage, Reflexology, Reiki, Relaxation,
Visualisation

Details: All therapies are available to clients on weekdays with
Acupuncture, Counselling, Cranio-Sacral Therapy,
Homeopathy, Reiki, Relaxation and Visualisation open to
carers, and Aromatherapy, Massage, Reflexology and Reiki
open to staff. Self referral and advance booking are required
for all therapies

Cost: All free of charge
There is a charge for staff who wish to have Aromatherapy,
Massage, Reflexology and Reiki. This is available through the
Stress Busters Service

Quality assurance: Patients and carers can self-refer, but can only access the complementary therapy service through a keyworker. All clients are seen by a keyworker on first appointment. Appointments for therapies are made in advance

Promotion: Complementary therapy service integrated with other services offered. Leaflets given by keyworkers in context of rehabilitation programme

BASIC (Brain & Spinal Injury Charity)

Sandra Buckley, Help line/Information Officer 0870 750 0000
(answering service: 5.30pm – 9.30am)
The Neurocare Centre, 554 Eccles New Road, Salford, Greater Manchester M5 2AL

Affiliated to Hope Hospital's Neurosciences Centre, BASIC offers patients and their families information and support. It specialises in supporting patients recovering from brain surgery and offers a sign-posting service to other neurological charities

Therapies: Aromatherapy, Counselling, Massage, Meditation, Reflexology, Relaxation, Visualisation

Details: All therapies are available to clients and carers on Mondays (including evenings), Tuesday mornings and Fridays. Aromatherapy, Massage and Reflexology are open to staff. Self referrals accepted for Aromatherapy, Massage, Meditation, Reflexology, Relaxation and Visualisation. Drop-in is available for Meditation, Relaxation and Visualisation. Book in advance for Aromatherapy, Counselling, Massage and Reflexology

Cost: Free of charge for Counselling
There is a fee for Aromatherapy, Massage, Meditation, Reflexology, Relaxation, Visualisation

Beechwood Cancer Care Centre

Samantha Parkin, Clinical Manager   **0161 476 0384**
Chelford Grove, Stockport, Greater Manchester SK3 8LS

A small charity providing psychosocial support to people and their carers, as soon as cancer is diagnosed, the Care Centre runs a 12-week programme which patients and carers attend once a week

Therapies:	Aromatherapy, Art Therapy, Massage, Music Therapy, Reflexology, Reiki, Relaxation, Visualisation
Details:	All therapies are available to clients and carers on weekdays on self referral. All therapies should be booked in advance (clients can also be referred by healthcare professionals)
Cost:	All free of charge. Patients and carers attending the 12-week programme receive complementary therapies free of charge. A fee-paying therapy service is also run (Friday 11.00-14.00) for the general public
Quality assurance:	Patients and carers are carefully assessed by an experienced therapist prior to any treatment. This process takes into account any existing medical conditions, treatments and side effects. Complementary therapists and nurse therapists must be qualified and have experience of working with cancer patients
Promotion:	Promote via health professionals, eg. GPs, clinical nurse specialists, Macmillan and district nurses; distribute leaflets and posters at main local hospitals; run talks at the centre for any interested, local groups, eg. Age Concern; attend local patients' and carers' information days; have used TV programmes to promote services and recruit volunteers

St Ann's Hospice

Ann Carter, Complementary Therapy Co-ordinator　　　　**0161 291 2912**

Peel Lane, Little Hulton, Worsley, Greater Manchester M38 0EL

Therapies:	Aromatherapy, Massage, Reflexology
Details:	All therapies are available to clients and carers. For inpatients, times vary according to demand – a reflexologist holds two afternoon sessions per week. All therapies are booked in advance; inpatients can self-refer or be referred by healthcare professionals; outpatients are referred though a healthcare professional
Cost:	All free of charge
Quality assurance:	The therapist will always screen for appropriateness. This applies especially to outpatients, while for inpatients, the therapists are all nurses who know the patients
Promotion:	Mainly through conversation and referrals from staff

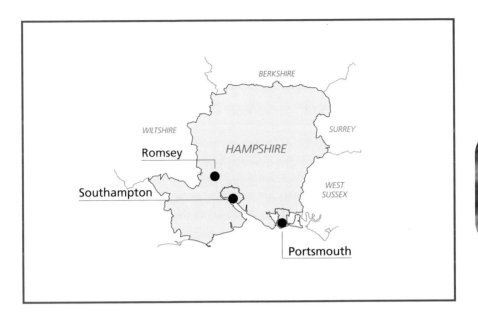

Complementary therapy services in

Hampshire

Portsmouth	• Macmillan Information & Support Centre
	• The Rowans (Portsmouth Area Hospice)
Romsey	• Cancer Care Society
Southampton	• Southampton University Hospitals Trust

Macmillan Information & Support Centre

Nicola Booth, Centre Manager   **023 9286 6408**
St Mary's Hospital, Milton Road, Portsmouth, Hampshire PO3 6AD

A purpose-built complementary therapy room within the Macmillan Support & Information Centre

Therapies:	Aromatherapy, Counselling, Massage, Indian Head (& Neck) Massage, Reflexology, Relaxation, Visualisation
Details:	All therapies are available to clients and carers on Monday afternoons, Wednesday afternoons, Thursdays and Fridays with Relaxation and Visualisation open to staff. Self referrals are accepted for all therapies; all can be booked in advance although Counselling and Relaxation are available on drop-in
Cost:	Please enquire
Quality assurance:	Vetted by complementary therapists for Aromatherapy, Reflexology and Massage. When asking for referral, patient/client is asked re contra-indications
Promotion:	Posters around hospital; leaflets; Aromatherapy/Reflexology being developed. Health professional referral; word of mouth; local media coverage

The Rowans (Portsmouth Area Hospice)

Ruth Summers, Matron   **023 9225 0001**
Purbrook Heath Road, Purbrook, Waterlooville, Portsmouth, Hampshire PO7 5RU

The Rowans operates a 19-bedded, specialist palliative care unit. It can also offer 16 places three days a week for specialist day care. It is an independent healthcare provider working in partnership with East Hants Primary Care Trust

Therapies:	Acupuncture, Aromatherapy, Massage, Reflexology, Relaxation, Visualisation
Details:	All therapies are available to clients on Monday, Wednesday and Thursday afternoons, with Relaxation and Visualisation

also open to carers, and Acupuncture, Aromatherapy, Massage and Reflexology open to staff. Professional referrals are required for all inpatient therapies with Massage also open to self referrals. Day care clients can self-refer for Aromatherapy, Massage, Acupuncture and Reflexology. Both inpatients and day care patients need to make bookings in advance for Aromatherapy, Massage and Reflexology.

Relaxation and Visualisation are provided by a clinical psychologist. Aromatherapy, Massage and Reflexology are provided by nurses and volunteers

Cost:	All free of charge
Quality assurance:	Assessment is made with the individual by therapists. Some written information is supplied. Evaluated and prescribed through care plan. Clinical psychologist provides Relaxation, Visualisation; physiotherapists provide Acupuncture
Promotion:	Leaflets; booklets

Cancer Care Society

01794 830300
11 The Cornmarket, Romsey, Hampshire SO51 8GB

Cancer Care is a registered charity with its Head Office in Romsey. It operates 5 walk-in centres in Wales (2), Norfolk (1) and Hampshire (2). Telephone contact/help available for any area

Therapies:	Aromatherapy, Counselling, Reflexology, Relaxation
Details:	All therapies are available to clients, carers and staff on weekdays. All are open to self referrals and require advance booking but Relaxation also open for drop-in. Clients and

carers can self-refer for support groups, which can be accessed either through the drop-in or booking service

Cost: All free of charge

Support groups for clients, carers and staff, are all free of charge

Quality assurance: Clearance from GP or consultant. Assessment session offered. Ongoing review of suitability. Explanation sheets available

Materials supplied: Our information library includes books and videos on complementary therapies

Promotion: Posters and leaflets in GPs' surgeries and in hospitals; media; specialist nurses; hospices

Southampton University Hospitals Trust

Sarah Chantler   **02380 475270**

Countess Mountbatten House, Moorgreen Hospital, Botley Road, West End, Southampton SO30 3JB

Countess Mountbatten House is Southampton's University Hospital Trust's specialist palliative care unit. This is a beacon service comprised of a 25 bedded inpatient unit, community service day care and education unit

Therapies: Acupuncture, Aromatherapy, Art Therapy, Nutritional Supplements, Reflexology, Reiki, Relaxation

Details: All therapies are available to clients through professional referral, with Aromatherapy, Reiki and Relaxation also open to staff. Advance booking is required

Cost: Free of charge, except for Aromatherapy for which staff pay a fee

Quality assurance: By the practitioners themselves. Medical approval is necessary for inpatients

Promotion: Via day care for day care patients and nurses for inpatients

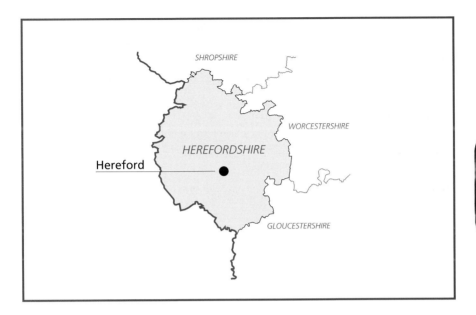

Complementary therapy services in
Herefordshire

Hereford   ● St Michael's Hospice

St Michael's Hospice

Jane Mason, Head of Nursing   **01432 851000**

Bartestree, Hereford, Herefordshire HR1 4HA

Therapies:	Acupuncture, Aromatherapy, Massage, Reflexology, Relaxation
Details:	All therapies are open to clients and carers on weekdays upon professional referral
Cost:	All free of charge
Promotion:	Leaflets

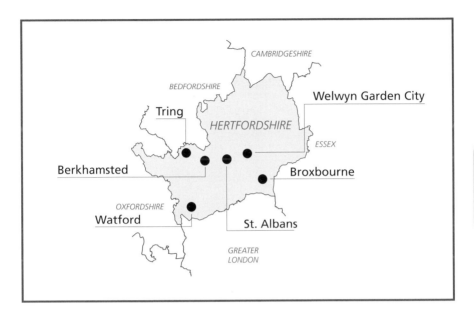

Complementary therapy services in

Hertfordshire

Berkhamsted	• Hospice of St Francis
Broxbourne	• Barnet & District Cancerlink
St Albans	• Grove House
Tring	• Iain Rennie Hospice at Home
Watford	• The Peace Hospice
Welwyn Garden City	• Isabel Hospice

Hospice of St Francis

Freda Magee, Complementary Therapy Co-ordinator　　　**01442 862960**
27 Shrublands Road, Berkhamsted, Hertfordshire HP4 3HX

The hospice provides inpatient care, home care, day care and bereavement counselling

Therapies:	Aromatherapy, Art Therapy, Counselling, Homeopathy, Massage, Meditation, Osteopathy, Reflexology, Relaxation, Visualisation
Details:	All therapies are available to inpatients Monday to Friday afternoons. Appointments are made individually for home care/bereavement counselling services. Additionally, Counselling is available for carers, and Aromatherapy, Massage and Reflexology are available to staff in evenings. Aromatherapy, Counselling, Massage, Meditation, Reflexology, Relaxation and Visualisation are available on self referral; Clients must be referred by a healthcare professional for Osteopathy, Art Therapy and Homeopathy. They may be referred by healthcare professionals for the other therapies
Cost:	All free of charge
Promotion:	Hospice leaflet; through information given by nurses on admission; through information given by home care team; through information given by bereavement counsellor; posters for staff

Barnet & District Cancerlink

Les Spicer, Chair　　　**01992 448056**
3 Borrell Close, Park Lane, Broxbourne, Hertfordshire EN10 7RD

Therapies:	Counselling, Massage, Reflexology, Reiki, Relaxation, Spiritual Healing
Details:	All therapies are available to clients and carers on Wednesday afternoons and every second Thursday of the month (18.00-

21.00). All therapies are available on self referral and drop-in

Cost: All free of charge
Materials supplied: Book library and cassettes
Promotion: Leaflets; posters; magazine; personal contact

Grove House

Carol Milsom, Team Secretary   **01727 897458**
Waverley Road, St. Albans, Hertfordshire AL3 5QX

Grove House offers a day hospice for cancer patients or those with life-threatening illness, plus outpatient services for patients at any stage of disease from pre-diagnosis onwards

Therapies: Aromatherapy, Art Therapy, Counselling, Massage, Reflexology, Reiki, Relaxation, Shiatsu
Details: All therapies are available on weekdays to clients and carers. Professional referral is required for Aromatherapy, Art Therapy, Massage, Reflexology, Reiki and Shiatsu; self referrals are accepted for Counselling and Relaxation. Book in advance for all therapies. Following drop-in, a patient is assessed by clinical nurse specialist
Cost: All free of charge
Materials supplied: Leaflets, cassettes
Promotion: Leaflets; posters; oncology clinic volunteers; Macmillan nurses/GPs; other palliative care/cancer care units

Iain Rennie Hospice at Home

Sue Jarvie   **01442 890444**
52a Western Road, Tring, Hertfordshire HP23 4BB

The hospice operates a 24-hour community specialist palliative care service known as hospice-at-home

Therapies:	Aromatherapy, Massage, Reflexology
Details:	All therapies are available to clients and carers on weekdays. Therapies are occasionally available in the evening and in emergencies on Saturday and Sunday. Professional referral is required for all therapies
Cost:	All free of charge
Quality assurance:	Full health questionnaire completed and medical background obtained from GP
Materials supplied:	Leaflets
Promotion:	Verbal explanation by a member of the nursing team when care planning is underway; leaflets are then made available if patient/carer is interested. Discuss therapies at formal meetings with primary healthcare team members

The Peace Hospice

Noel Ratcliffe, Director of Nursing   **01923 330330**
Peace Drive, off Cassiobury Drive, Watford, Hertfordshire WD17 3PH

Therapies:	Aromatherapy, Counselling, Massage, Reflexology
Details:	All therapies are available to clients on weekdays, except Fridays (plus Monday to Friday evenings) with Counselling also available to carers. Self referrals are accepted for all therapies and Counselling may be booked in advance (clients can be referred by health professionals)
Cost:	All free of charge
Quality assurance:	Before treatment, a referral form detailing patient's condition is completed and practitioner discusses therapy with client
Promotion:	By describing to clients at admission assessment interview. By communicating to nursing staff and duty therapists

Isabel Hospice

Pam Harvey, Director of Nursing   **01707 330686**

Griffin House, Watchmead, Welwyn Garden City, Hertfordshire AL7 1LT

Therapies:	Aromatherapy, Art Therapy, Counselling, Massage, Indian Head (& Neck) Massage, Music Therapy, Reflexology, Reiki, Relaxation, Visualisation
Details:	All therapies are available to clients and carers on Mondays, Tuesdays, Thursdays and Fridays, with morning and evening sessions available on Wednesdays. Massage, Reflexology and Reiki are also available to staff. Aromatherapy, Counselling, Massage, Indian Head (& Neck) Massage, Reflexology, Reiki, Relaxation and Visualisation are open to self referrals or can be referred by a healthcare professional. All therapies should be booked in advance
Cost:	All free of charge
Quality assurance:	Complementary therapies are offered as a supportive measure, not as a treatment. Discussion of desired or appropriate therapy is made on initial contact, always with patient's condition taken into account. Manner of all therapies is of a most gentle nature. Full understanding of what each therapy is and how it is carried out
Promotion:	Specialist nurses employed by hospice; information package; breast, respiratory, colon clinic nurses at area hospital; drop-in day at day hospice; carers group at day hospice. Word of mouth by staff at all hospice sites

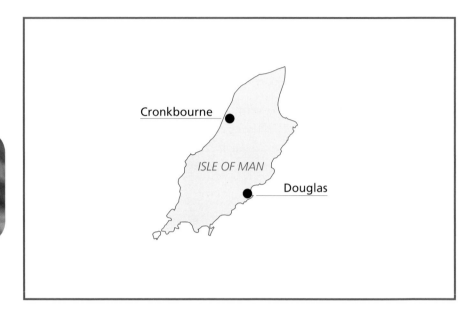

Complementary therapy services in

Isle of Man

Cronkbourne	• Manx Cancer Help Association
Douglas	• St Bridget's Hospice

Manx Cancer Help Association

Mrs Eve Berridge, Care Co-ordinator　　　　　　　　　**01624 679544**
The Lisa Lowe Centre, Old School House, Cronkbourne, Isle of Man　IM4 4QH

Started in 1983, the association now employs an administrator and a counsellor/befriender. Most patients self-refer, and most work with them takes place in their homes. Follow-up bereavement visits are also offered where appropriate

Therapies:	Counselling, Meditation, Nutritional Programmes, Relaxation, Spiritual Healing, Nutritional Supplements, Visualisation
Details:	All therapies are available to clients and carers on weekdays (including evenings) and on Saturday mornings, with Counselling also available to staff. All therapies are open to self referrals and should be booked in advance
Cost:	All free of charge
Quality assurance:	Care co-ordinator attended courses for 18 years at Bristol Cancer Help Centre and Manchester University's conference of Cancer Self-Help Groups. Initial visit to patient and carer is to discuss their needs and work out suitable protocol for them
Materials supplied:	Library, videos, CDs, cassettes, CancerBACUP literature and information from Bristol Cancer Help Centre and New Approaches to Cancer
Promotion:	Leaflets in local hospitals; leaflets in GPs' surgeries; free, weekly advertisement in Manx free newspaper

St Bridget's Hospice

Dr B Harris, Medical Director　　　　　　　　　　　**01624 834159**
Hospice Care (Isle of Man), Dorothy Pantin House, Kensington Road, Douglas, Isle of Man　IM1 3PE

Therapies:	Acupuncture, Aromatherapy, Counselling, Massage, Reflexology, Relaxation

ENGLAND Isle of Man

Details: Available to clients, carers and staff on weekdays (including
                     evenings) and on Saturdays. Professional referral and advance
                     booking are required
Cost: All free of charge
Quality assurance: Comprehensive referral form. Assessment by Medical Director.
                     Regular review of those being treated
Promotion: Leaflets; website; posters; advice by other professionals

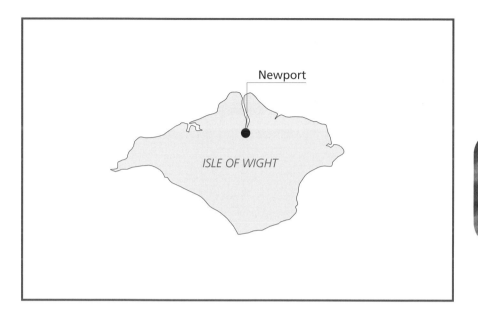

Complementary therapy services in
Isle of Wight

Newport
- Earl Mountbatten Hospice
- Isle of Wight NHS Healthcare Trust

Earl Mountbatten Hospice

Anne Tyrrell   **01983 529511**
Halberry Lane, Newport, Isle of Wight PO30 2ER

The Earl Mountbatten Hospice covers the whole Isle of Wight population of 128,000 as there are no other specialist palliative care units

Therapies:	Acupuncture, Aromatherapy, Counselling, Massage, Reflexology, Relaxation, Therapeutic Touch, Visualisation
Details:	Acupuncture, Aromatherapy, Counselling, Massage, Reflexology, Relaxation, Visualisation are open to clients on weekday afternoons, with Counselling and Therapeutic Touch also offered to carers. All therapies require professional referral (Massage also open to self referral). All therapies should be booked in advance (Therapeutic Touch open to drop-in)
Cost:	All free of charge
Quality assurance:	Medical staff aware of patient's condition and this is well documented. A complementary therapy resource person, who is a trained reflexologist and masseuse, checks for contra-indications. This person refers patients to trained voluntary therapists as appropriate. If therapists are in any doubt, they will refer back to medical staff or the complementary therapist resource person
Promotion:	Via nursing staff or the resource person for complementary therapies

Isle of Wight NHS Healthcare Trust

Andrew Gallini, Lead Cancer Nurse   **01983 534972**
St Mary's Hospital, Parkhurst Road, Newport, Isle of Wight PO30 1NZ

Therapies:	Aromatherapy, Massage, Reflexology, Relaxation, Yoga
Details:	Relaxation is available to clients with cancer who may self

refer (contact for details of availability) and Aromatherapy, Massage, Reflexology, Relaxation and Yoga are available to staff

Cost: Free of charge for clients for Relaxation
There is a fee for staff for Aromatherapy, Massage, Reflexology, Yoga.

Book in advance: Relaxation

Promotion: Leaflets; posters; internal e-mails; via breast care unit

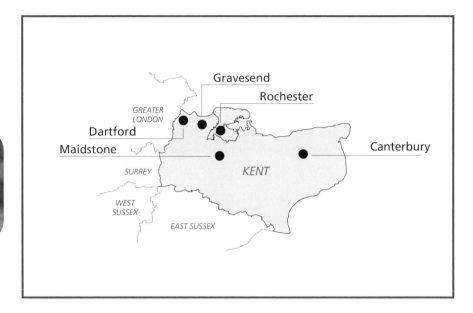

Complementary therapy services in

Kent

Canterbury	● Cancer Information Support & Counselling Service
	● Pilgrims Hospice in East Kent
Dartford	● The Ellenor Foundation
Gravesend	● The Lions Hospice
Maidstone	● The Bearsted Holistic Cancer & Stress Self-Help &
Rochester	● Wisdom Hospice

Cancer Information Support & Counselling Service

Elizabeth Taylor   01227 864045
Supportive Therapies Bungalow, Oncology Dept, Kent & Canterbury Hospital,
Ethelbert Road, Canterbury, Kent CT1 3NG

Therapies:	Aromatherapy, Counselling, Massage, Reflexology, Relaxation, Shiatsu
Details:	All therapies are available to clients Monday to Thursday and Friday mornings. Counselling is also open to carers and staff. All therapies are open to self referrals and should be advance booked
Cost:	All free of charge for first ten sessions; charge made thereafter
Promotion:	Leaflets; word of mouth referrals by nurses, radiographers etc

Pilgrims Hospice in East Kent

Dr Anthony M Smith, Medical Director   01227 459700
56 London Road, Canterbury, Kent CT2 8JA

Hospices in Ashford, Canterbury and Margate provide 59 inpatient specialist palliative
care beds for people with advanced/progressive/incurable disease. There is a day
centre at each unit and palliative advisory team of 16 specialist community nurses

Therapies:	Aromatherapy, Art Therapy, Counselling, Massage, Reflexology
Details:	All therapies are available to clients on weekday afternoons (Counselling is available from 09.00 to 17.00) with Counselling available to carers and Aromatherapy, Counselling, Massage and Reflexology open to staff. All therapies require professional referral (clients can self-refer for Counselling) and advance booking
Cost:	Please enquire
Quality assurance:	Provided by the therapist

Materials supplied:	Entry in hospice handbook which is given to all patients on admission
Promotion:	Personal recommendations made in the day centre and ward; referral of patients from the multidisciplinary team; there is an entry in the hospice handbook which is given to each patient; a leaflet regarding support facilities is given to staff

The Ellenor Foundation

Cate Masheder   01322 221315
East Hill, Dartford, Kent DA1 1SA

A hospice home care team is run from a purpose-built building, but there is no inpatient unit

Therapies:	Aromatherapy, Counselling, Massage, Reflexology
Details:	All therapies are available to clients, carers and staff on weekdays. Self referrals are accepted; all therapies to be advance booked
Cost:	All free of charge
Quality assurance:	Assessment by individual practitioner
Promotion:	Clinical nurse specialists offer to patient/carer

The Lions Hospice

01474 320007
Coldharbour Road, Northfleet, Gravesend, Kent DA11 7HQ

The Lions is a hospice with 12 inpatient beds and 80 places for day therapy per week

Therapies:	Acupuncture, Aromatherapy, Art Therapy, Counselling, Drama Therapy, Massage, Music Therapy, Reflexology
Details:	All therapies are available to clients on Mondays, Thursdays (including evening) and Friday mornings. Aromatherapy,

Massage and Reflexology are open to carers and staff.
Professional referral is required

Cost: Therapies for patients are free of charge
Therapies for staff are for a fee.
A donation is accepted from carers, but is not a requirement

Quality assurance: If patients do self-refer, a check is made with their GP before proceeding (no procedures are in place yet). Each therapist completes his or her own medical assessment before treating

Promotion: Day therapy leaflet; inpatient leaflet

The Bearsted Holistic Cancer & Stress Self-Help & Support Group

Kathleen Wingrove, Founder   **01622 730133**
Lavender Cottage, Bearsted Road, Maidstone, Kent ME14 5LD

Independent and self-supporting, the Group rents the local Friends Meeting House which is spacious, modern and has all the necessary facilities, including parking. Registered with Maidstone Voluntary Bureau and the Bristol Cancer Help Centre

Therapies: Art Therapy, Bach Flower Remedies (or Flower Essences), Counselling, Cranio-Sacral Therapy, Massage, Meditation, Reflexology, Reiki, Relaxation, Spiritual Healing, Therapeutic Touch, Visualisation

Details: All therapies are available to clients, carers and staff on the first Tuesday (10.30–13.30) and second Friday (20.00-22.00) of each month. All open to self referral and drop-in

Cost: All free of charge

Quality assurance: Therapists are trained and know when their therapies are contra-indicated. The group works together and to some degree, clients choose the therapy that they find helps them the most

Materials supplied: Own Relaxation/Visualisation tape, books, videos, tapes, music and cancer magazines

Promotion: Leaflets; posters; registered with local hospital, CancerBACUP, Cancerlink, Bristol Cancer Help Centre who refer patients. Give talks to hospitals etc

Wisdom Hospice

Mrs Margaret Simpson, Senior Nurse Manager   **01634 830456**

Thames Gateway NHS Trust, St William's Way, Rochester, Kent ME1 2NU

Part of the Trust's palliative care directorate – day hospice, community team, inpatient unit, therapists and social work teams. All operate jointly from one base to provide seamless, specialist palliative care to residents of Medway & Swale

Therapies: Aromatherapy, Art Therapy, Counselling, Hypnotherapy/Hypnosis, Massage, Indian Head (& Neck) Massage, Music Therapy, Reflexology, Reiki, Relaxation

Details: All therapies are available to clients on weekday afternoons and Thursday evenings with Counselling open to carers, and Aromatherapy, Counselling, Massage and Reflexology available to staff. Aromatherapy, Counselling, Massage, Reflexology and Reiki by self and professional referral. Hypnotherapy/Hypnosis, Music Therapy and Relaxation by professional referral only. Relaxation to be booked in advance

Cost: Free of charge for Counselling, Relaxation
There is a fee for Aromatherapy, Massage, Reflexology

Quality assurance: Carry out holistic assessment of patient

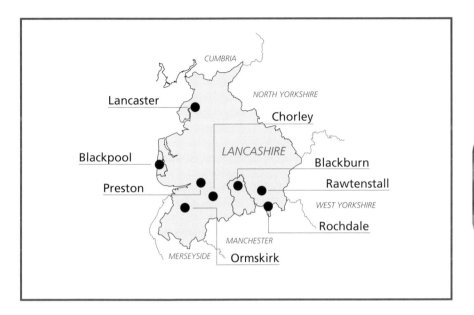

Complementary therapy services in

Lancashire

Blackburn	• East Lancashire Hospice
Blackpool	• Blackpool Victoria Hospital NHS Trust
	• Cancer VIVE
	• Trinity Palliative Care Services
Chorley	• Derian House Children's Hospice
Lancaster	• CancerCare (North Lancashire and South Lakeland)
	• Royal Lancaster Infirmary
	• St John's Hospice
Ormskirk	• Southport & Ormskirk District General Hospital
Preston	• Cancer Help Preston Ltd
Rochdale	• Macmillan Nursing Service
Rawtenstall	• East Lancashire Integrated Health Care Centre

East Lancashire Hospice

Community Macmillan Team
Park Lee Road, Blackburn, Lancashire BB1 3NY

From January 2002, the Macmillan team will be based at the East Lancashire Hospice, but will remain a community team

Therapies:	Aromatherapy, Reflexology, Reiki
Details:	Available on Mondays to clients and carers on professional referral
Cost:	All free of charge
Quality assurance:	Patients attend day therapy unit and are assessed by therapists
Promotion:	Discuss during home visits

Blackpool Victoria Hospital NHS Trust

Sister Maria Ronson   01253 306836
Haemotology/Oncology Department, Whinney Heys Road, Blackpool, Lancashire FY3 8NR

Complementary therapy service started in January 2002

Therapies:	Aromatherapy, Massage, Relaxation
Details:	Available to clients on Thursdays by self referral and advance booking (can be referred by healthcare professional)
Cost:	All free of charge
Quality assurance:	Policy with specific criteria set for patients: who can/cannot receive therapies
Promotion:	Posters; leaflets

Cancer VIVE

Jackie Dimuantes, Secretary   **01253 357424**
7 Waller Avenue, Bispham, Blackpool, Lancashire FY2 9EL

A self-help group using a holistic approach

Therapies:	Aromatherapy, Art Therapy, Counselling, Massage, Meditation, Reflexology, Reiki, Relaxation, Spiritual Healing, Therapeutic Touch, Visualisation
Details:	All therapies are available to clients, carers and staff one Saturday every month on self referral. Clients can be referred by a healthcare professional for Massage, Reflexology and Aromatherapy
Cost:	All free of charge
Quality assurance:	Doctor's permission is sought for hands-on therapies. Therapists are qualified and insured
Materials supplied:	Books, cassettes
Promotion:	Posters; leaflets; informed on arrival; information in library

Trinity Palliative Care Services

Beryl Porter, Palliative Care Nurse Co-ordinator   **01253 358881**
Low Moor Road, Blackpool, Lancashire FY2 0BG

Therapies:	Art Therapy, Counselling, Music Therapy, Relaxation, Nutritional Supplements
Details:	All therapies are available to clients on weekdays (Counselling is also available Monday to Thursday evenings). Additionally, Counselling open to carers and staff. Professional referral is required for Art Therapy, Music Therapy, Relaxation and Nutritional Supplements with Counselling on self referral. Counselling to be advance booked
Cost:	Please enquire
Promotion:	Information leaflets and Information service

Derian House Children's Hospice

Joyce Dilworth, Nursery Nurse   **01257 233300**
Chancery Road, Astley Village, Chorley, Lancashire PR7 1DH

A children's hospice

Therapies:	Aromatherapy, Massage, Reflexology, Reiki
Details:	All therapies are available to clients, carers and staff on self referral (contact for details of availability)
Cost:	Please enquire
Promotion:	Leaflets; word of mouth

CancerCare (North Lancashire and South Lakeland)

T Dougan, Head of Complementary Therapies   **01524 381820**
Slynedales, Slyne Road, Lancaster, Lancashire LA2 6ST

Therapies:	Alexander Technique, Aromatherapy, Art Therapy, Counselling, Massage, Relaxation, Visualisation, Yoga
Details:	All therapies are available to clients and carers on weekdays (including Tuesday evenings) with Counselling, Relaxation and Yoga open to staff. Professional referral and advance booking required
Cost:	All free of charge
Quality assurance:	Assessment made when referral received
Materials supplied:	CancerBACUP's complementary therapy booklets and information available
Promotion:	Leaflets; posters/displays on oncology units; talking to professionals; use of the press

Royal Lancaster Infirmary

Jane Kerr   **01524 583703**
Ashton Road, Lancaster, Lancashire LA1 4RP

District General Hospital providing access to complementary therapies via CancerCare at Slynedales. Currently, the service is not available to inpatients

Therapies:	Aromatherapy, Art Therapy, Counselling, Massage, Relaxation, Visualisation
Details:	All therapies are available to clients and carers on self referral (contact T Dougan on 01524 381820). Advance booking required
Cost:	All free of charge
Quality assurance:	An assessment process is undertaken by therapists prior to commencing a course of therapy
Promotion:	Informing verbally; leaflets; open days

St John's Hospice

Clive Shelley, General Manager   **01524 382538**
Slyne Road, Lancaster, Lancashire LA2 6AW

A hospice providing inpatient care, day care and bereavement support for North Lancashire and South Lakeland

Therapies:	Aromatherapy, Art Therapy, Counselling, Massage, Yoga
Details:	Aromatherapy, Art Therapy, Counselling and Massage are available to clients on professional referral on weekday afternoons except Wednesday. Yoga is available to staff on self referral
Cost:	All free of charge
	Complementary therapies are provided by Cancercare
Quality assurance:	Discussion with therapist. 'Hand-over' protocol
Promotion:	Talking to patients; advertising in day care literature

Southport & Ormskirk District General Hospital

Complementary Therapy Centre   **01695 656100**

Ormskirk & District General Hospital, Wigan Road, Ormskirk, Lancashire L39 2AZ

The complementary therapy centre is a service for NHS staff free of charge, but also accepts patient referrals only from consultants based at Southport and Ormskirk hospitals

Therapies:	Aromatherapy, Massage, Reflexology, Reiki, Relaxation
Details:	All therapies are primarily available to staff, but also to clients and carers from Tuesday to Friday on professional referral. All booked in advance. Staff can self-refer for Relaxation, Aromatherapy, Massage, Reflexology and Reiki
Cost:	Please enquire
Quality assurance:	Professional experienced staff in complementary therapy centre. Leaflets detail side effects which may be caused by complementary therapies
Materials supplied:	Literature
Promotion:	Leaflets and posters; e-mail; word of mouth; consultant referrals; occupational health

Cancer Help Preston Ltd

Mrs Margaret O'Donoghue SRN SCM   **01772 793344**

Vine House Cancer Day Centre, 22 Cromwell Road, Ribbleton, Preston, Lancashire PR2 6YB

A day centre providing advice, information, complementary and social therapies

Therapies:	Aromatherapy, Art Therapy, Counselling, Massage, Meditation, Reflexology, Reiki, Relaxation, Spiritual Healing, Visualisation
Details:	All therapies are available on weekdays to clients and carers on self referral. (Aromatherapy, Massage and Relaxation are occasionally open to staff.) All therapies booked in advance but Counselling also available on drop-in

Cost:	All free of charge
Quality assurance:	All patients requesting therapies undertake detailed assessment, including medical history. Assessment by registered general nurse with oncology/palliative care experience. All therapists, who are fully qualified in their own field, assess patient prior to commencing therapy
Materials supplied:	Leaflets, cassettes, books, videos
Promotion:	Leaflets, posters, newspaper, radio, word of mouth, video. Close liaison with community and hospital healthcare teams, particularly hospital oncology clinics

Macmillan Nursing Service

Macmillan Nursing Team   **01706 651967**
Milnrow Health Centre, Stonefield Street, Milnrow, Rochdale, Lancashire OL16 4HZ

Therapies:	Aromatherapy, Massage, Reflexology, Relaxation
Details:	All therapies are available to clients and carers by professional referral on the last Wednesday morning of each month – the Breast Care Group also meets at this time. Therapies are also available at a local resource centre by appointment on Friday afternoons. Home visits for complementary therapies can be arranged with clients
Cost:	Nutritional supplements are available with a prescription
Quality assurance:	Assessment by therapist. Verbal discussion with patient
Materials supplied:	Relaxation tapes
Promotion:	Verbal information due to time limitations; involved with breast cancer support group

East Lancashire Integrated Health Care Centre

Helen Hill   **01706 240080**
Cribden House, Rossendale Hospital, Rawtenstall, Lancashire BB4 6NE

Therapies:	Aromatherapy, Counselling, Hypnotherapy/Hypnosis, Massage, Meditation, Neuro-Linguistic Programming, Psychotherapy, Reflexology, Reiki, Relaxation, Visualisation
Details:	All therapies are available to clients and carers on weekdays by self referral (clients can be referred for complementary therapies by healthcare professionals)
Cost:	Please enquire
Quality assurance:	Policy in place
Materials supplied:	Leaflets
Promotion:	Leaflets

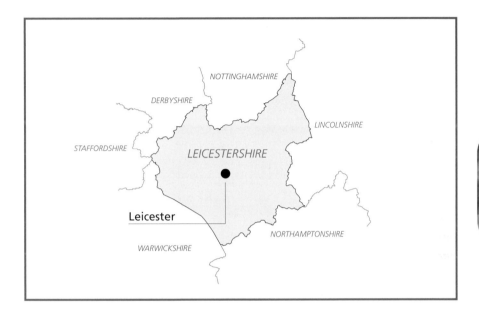

Complementary therapy services in

Leicestershire

Leicester
- Coping With Cancer in Leicestershire & Rutland
- The Leicestershire and Rutland Hospice (LOROS)

Coping With Cancer in Leicestershire and Rutland

Joanna Hamilton, Charity Manager   **0116 2230055**

Helen Webb House, 35 Westleigh Road, Fosse Road South, Leicester, Leicestershire LE3 0HH

A community-based, support centre for cancer patients, their families and friends

Therapies:	Aromatherapy, Art Therapy, Counselling, Massage, Indian Head (& Neck) Massage, Reflexology, Reiki, Relaxation, Visualisation
Details:	All therapies are available to clients on weekdays and alternate Tuesday evenings by self referral, with Aromatherapy, Counselling, Massage, Indian Head (& Neck) Massage, Reflexology, Reiki, Relaxation and Visualisation also open to carers. Advance booking is required
Cost:	Please enquire
Quality assurance:	Policy for the provision of complementary therapies. Complementary treatment sheet. Referral form
Materials supplied:	Booklet with description of each therapy
Promotion:	Booklet; leaflets; linkworkers; clinical nurse specialists

The Leicestershire and Rutland Hospice (LOROS)

Diane Briscombe   **0116 2313771**

Groby Road, Leicester, Leicestershire LE3 9QE

A 29-bedded unit with a separate day centre which can cater for 25 places daily

Therapies:	Aromatherapy, Art Therapy, Counselling, Massage, Reflexology, Reiki, Relaxation, Visualisation
Details:	All therapies are available to clients and carers on Tuesday afternoons/evenings, Wednesdays and Fridays, with

Aromatherapy, Massage, Reflexology, Reiki, Relaxation and Visualisation also open to staff. Professional referral is required for Aromatherapy, Massage, Reflexology, Reiki, Relaxation and Visualisation; self referrals accepted for Art Therapy and Counselling

Cost: All free of charge

Promotion: Currently developing a leaflet

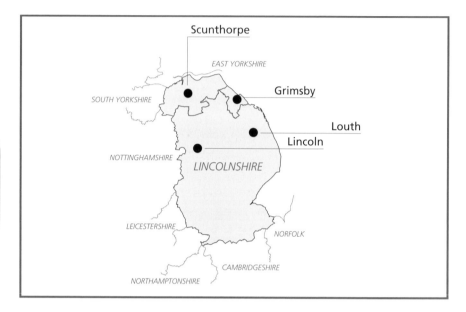

Complementary therapy services in

Lincolnshire

Grimsby	● Fresh Fields Breast Awareness Support Group
Lincoln	● St Barnabas Hospice
Louth	● Louth Breastcare Support Group
Scunthorpe	● Lindsey Lodge Hospice

Fresh Fields Breast Awareness Support Group

Margaret Johnson   **01472 506 993**
64a Welholme Avenue, Grimsby DN32 0PN

Fresh Fields is a dedicated breast care centre

Therapies:	Aromatherapy, Counselling, Massage, Reflexology, Relaxation
Details:	All therapies are available to clients on Monday mornings (and Relaxation is also available on Wednesday mornings) through professional referral. Self referral is also accepted for Relaxation. Counselling is also open to carers and staff. Book in advance for Bowen Technique. This is a pilot service unable to accommodate many referrals
Cost:	All free of charge; a charge is made for some Relaxation
Quality assurance:	Detailed information is given in referral. An assessment is undertaken by the therapist prior to any procedure being carried out
Promotion:	Leaflets; word of mouth

St Barnabas Hospice

Sarah Dunn   **01522 518209**
Hawthorn Road, Cherry Willingham, Lincoln, Lincolnshire LN3 4JR

Complementary therapies available three days a week in day hospice

Therapies:	Aromatherapy, Art Therapy, Massage, Reflexology, Relaxation
Details:	All therapies are available to clients on Tuesdays to Thursdays through self referral (Aromatherapy and Massage are

available when qualified nurse/therapist on duty)
Aromatherapy, Massage and Reflexology are also open to
staff. Relaxation and a pilot study in Reflexology are starting in
2002

Cost: Please enquire

Materials supplied: Leaflets

Promotion: Leaflets; explanation given in person by therapist or nursing
staff

Louth Breastcare Support Group

Mrs J F Loveley, Chairperson　　　　　　　　　　　**01507 602543**

Meeting Place, The Green Room, Louth Salvation Army Church, Church Street, Louth,
Lincolnshire

A friendly setting where people, and friends/carers, can receive emotional support.
Complementary therapies are provided only at group meetings.

Therapies: Aromatherapy, Art Therapy, Counselling, Herbal Remedies,
Reflexology, Relaxation, Nutritional Supplements

Details: Available on Monday evenings to clients and carers. Clients
can access therapies by belonging to the support group

Cost: Please enquire

Materials supplied: Tapes from New Approaches to Cancer are lent, when
supplied to the group

Promotion: At meetings where trained people give advice to those who
have/had cancer

Lindsey Lodge Hospice

Mrs Alison Tindall, Hospice Director   **01724 270835**

Burringham Road, Scunthorpe, Lincolnshire DN17 2AA

Lindsey Lodge is a hospice offering day care to 14 patients and a 10-bedded inpatient unit opened in February 2002

Therapies:	Aromatherapy, Art Therapy, Massage, Relaxation, Visualisation
Details:	Available to clients with professional referrals on weekdays
Cost:	Please enquire
Quality assurance:	Policy document
Materials supplied:	Patient library of useful information
Promotion:	In-house information

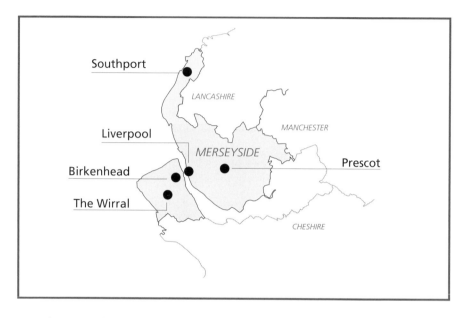

Complementary therapy services in

Merseyside

Birkenhead	• Wirral Holistic Therapeutic Cancer Care
Liverpool	• Liverpool Cancer Support Centre
	• Marie Curie Centre - Liverpool
	• North Mersey Community NHS Trust
	• Royal Liverpool University Hospital
	• Sefton Cancer Support Group
	• Woodlands Day Hospice
Prescot	• Lilac Centre
	• Willowbrook Hospice
Southport	• Queenscourt Hospice
The Wirral	• Claire House Children's Hospice
	• Clatterbridge Centre for Oncology
	• St John's Hospice in Wirral

Wirral Holistic Therapeutic Cancer Care

Mrs D Crowther, Chief Executive   **0151 604 7316**

St Catherine's Hospital, Church Road, Birkenhead, Merseyside CH42 0LQ

Therapies:	Acupuncture, Aromatherapy, Chiropractic, Counselling, Cranio-Sacral Therapy, Massage, Meditation, Nutritional Programmes, Reflexology, Reiki, Relaxation, Shiatsu, Spiritual Healing, Therapeutic Touch, Visualisation
Details:	All therapies are available to clients on weekdays (including Tuesday evenings) with Counselling, Nutritional Programmes, Reiki and Spiritual Healing also open to carers, and Counselling open to staff. All are by self referral and should be booked in advance or can be referred by healthcare professional
Cost:	All free of charge

Liverpool Cancer Support Centre

Mrs Sheila Keatley, Chairperson   **0151 726 8934**

21 Aigburth Road, Liverpool, Merseyside L17 4JR

The Centre is a purpose-built facility with disabled access and facilities. It is run by people who have been affected by cancer and operates with a strong ethos for self-help and user involvement

Therapies:	Acupuncture, Aromatherapy, Art Therapy, Massage, Reflexology, Relaxation
Details:	All therapies are available to clients and carers on Tuesdays and Thursdays by self referral. Book in advance for all except Art Therapy
Cost:	All free of charge
Quality assurance:	Consent form must be signed by patient's doctor before Aromatherapy, Massage and Reflexology commence
Materials supplied:	Books, videos, cassettes, library
Promotion:	Leaflets; posters

Marie Curie Cancer Care

Elaine Rosser   **0151 801 1400 x 1480/1453**

Marie Curie Cancer Care, Speke Road, Woolton, Liverpool, Merseyside L25 8QA

Currently offering Aromatherapy/Reflexology to Liverpool residents in the community. This is funded through the New Opportunities Fund for three years to 2003

Therapies:	Acupuncture, Aromatherapy, Massage, Reflexology, Relaxation
Details:	All therapies are available to clients on professional referral. Operates Monday and Tuesday afternoons, Wednesday mornings, Thursday afternoons and Fridays at community clinics for Liverpool residents only. Complementary therapy clinics are held in the Marie Curie Centre, Liverpool on Mondays, Thursdays and Fridays, 09.00-17.00. Advance booking required
Cost:	All free of charge
Quality assurance:	Information sheets are available for patients pre- and post-Aromatherapy/Reflexology
Promotion:	Leaflets to GPs, Trusts, information centres; posters; attending primary care group meetings

North Mersey Community NHS Trust

Mrs Anne Bainbridge, Clinic Manager   **0151 228 6808**

Depart. of Homoeopathic Medicine, Old Swan Health Centre, St Oswalds Street, Liverpool, Merseyside L13 2BY

Therapies:	Homeopathy, Iscador
Details:	Available to new patients through professional referral on Wednesdays and Thursday afternoons (follow-up visits are on other days). Homeopathy is also available to carers
Cost:	All free of charge
Materials supplied:	Leaflets
Promotion:	Information held by GPs

Royal Liverpool University Hospital

Pam Shepherd, Complementary Therapy Nurse Specialist		**0151 706 2000**
		x3249

Supportive Therapy Unit (c/o 8B Registry Room), Prescot Street, Liverpool, Merseyside L7 8XP

Therapies:	Aromatherapy, Massage, Reflexology, Relaxation, Therapeutic Touch, Visualisation
Details:	All therapies are available to clients on Mondays, Thursday mornings and Friday afternoons through professional referral
Cost:	All free of charge
Quality assurance:	Referral only via hospital's specialist nurses or medical team
Materials supplied:	Lend relaxation tapes; information on use of Aromatherapy if appropriate
Promotion:	Leaflets

Sefton Cancer Support Group

Mrs Barbara Eastwood, Chairperson	**01704 879352**

'Ashurst', 19 Duke Street, Formby, Liverpool, Merseyside L37 4AN

The group is self-contained, with its own rooms in a large house

Therapies:	Acupuncture, Reflexology, Relaxation, Spiritual Healing
Details:	Available to clients and carers on self referral: Tuesday mornings Spiritual Healing; Wednesday mornings Reflexology; Thursday mornings Acupuncture. Book in advance for Reflexology and Spiritual Healing; drop-in for Acupuncture and Relaxation
Cost:	Fee charged
Quality assurance:	All clients interviewed by accredited therapists before treatment. If therapists have any concerns, they are asked to speak to patient's consultant
Promotion:	Leaflets; word of mouth

Woodlands Day Hospice

Tilly Reid, Clinical Manager   **0151 529 2299**

UHA Campus, Longmoor Lane, Fazakerley, Liverpool, Merseyside L9 7LA

Woodlands Day Hospice is situated in the gounds of University Hospital Aintree, in North Liverpool, serving a population of 320,000

Therapies:	Acupuncture, Aromatherapy, Counselling, Massage, Reflexology, Relaxation, Visualisation
Details:	All therapies are available to clients on weekdays through professional referral with Aromatherapy, Reflexology and Relaxation available to carers
Cost:	Please enquire
Quality assurance:	Clinical protocols have been drawn up for Aromatherapy, Reflexology and Acupuncture. These are reviewed annually
Promotion:	The hospice produces its own leaflets for Aromatherapy, Reflexology and Acupuncture explaining what they are and how people may benefit from them. Talks on complementary therapies are regularly given, including demonstrations, as part of the hospice group therapy sessions

Lilac Centre

Gillian Levey/Shirlie Deveney   **0151 430 1687**

Whiston Hospital, Prescot, Merseyside WA9

The centre provides chemotherapy treatment, haematology treatment and complementary therapies. It provides patients with holistic support in a comfortable, relaxed environment

Therapies:	Aromatherapy, Counselling, Reflexology, Relaxation, Visualisation
Details:	All therapies are available to clients and carers by self referral (also professional referral for Aromatherapy, Counselling, Reflexology and Visualisation) on weekdays with Counselling

and Relaxation open to staff. All therapies can be advance
booked but Counselling is also available on drop-in

Cost:	All free of charge
Quality assurance:	Leaflet information. Assessment discussion. Consultation with nursing/medical staff
Promotion:	Leaflets and posters, word of mouth

Willowbrook Hospice

Norman Dunsby   **0151 430 8736**
Portico Lane, Prescot, Merseyside L34 1QT

Therapies:	Aromatherapy, Art Therapy, Counselling, Massage, Music Therapy, Nutritional Programmes, Reflexology, Relaxation, Nutritional Supplements, Therapeutic Touch, Visualisation
Details:	All therapies are available to clients Tuesdays to Thursdays with Aromatherapy, Counselling, Massage, Relaxation and Visualisation also open to carers and Aromatherapy, Massage, Reflexology, Relaxation, Therapeutic Touch and Visualisation open to staff. Professional referral and advance booking are required
Cost:	All free of charge
Quality assurance:	Chemotherapy and side effects discussed with medical team before any treatments given
Materials supplied:	Audiotapes available through health shops, CancerBACUP leaflets
Promotion:	Leaflets; through referral criteria to healthcare professionals

Queenscourt Hospice

Dr Karen Groves, Medical Director   **01704 544645**
Town Lane, Southport, Merseyside PR8 6RE

Queenscourt is an independent, voluntary hospice providing multiprofessional, palliative
assessment and management in inpatient, day therapy and outpatient settings

Therapies:	Acupuncture, Aromatherapy, Art Therapy, Counselling, Herbal Remedies, Massage, Music Therapy, Nutritional Programmes, Reflexology, Relaxation, Nutritional Supplements, Therapeutic Touch, Visualisation
Details:	Available to clients Tuesday to Friday by professional referral. Patients and carers only access services by referral from a GP or hospital consultant. (Referrals are not accepted from anyone else or for therapies in isolation.) Psychological support is provided through Counselling; every inpatient is prescribed Nutritional Supplements when medically necessary
Cost:	Please enquire
Quality assurance:	All therapies are given under medical supervision and subject to team evaluation

Claire House Children's Hospice

Deirdre Martin, Physiotherapist   **0151 334 4626**
Clatterbridge Road, Bebington, The Wirral, Merseyside CH48 2JL

A children's hospice

Therapies:	Aromatherapy, Counselling, Massage, Music Therapy
Details:	Aromatherapy, Massage and Music Therapy are available to clients and carers from Tuesday to Thursday (also on Mondays, Fridays, Saturdays and Sundays depending on shift patterns) with Aromatherapy, Counselling and Massage also open to staff. Counselling is available by booking and drop-in. Children must be referred by a healthcare professional for Aromatherapy and Massage; carers, however, can self-refer for these therapies. Counselling and Music Therapy are offered through self-referral
Cost:	All free of charge
Quality assurance:	All children have a care plan. All children have an

Aromatherapy plan, on which all contra-indications and health problems are charted

Promotion: Letters to families; word of mouth

Clatterbridge Centre for Oncology

Complementary Therapy Co-ordinator   **0151 334 1155**

Clatterbridge Road, Bebington, The Wirral, Merseyside CH63 4JY

An oncology centre providing radiotherapy and chemotherapy for both inpatients and outpatients

Therapies: Aromatherapy

Details: Available to clients on Tuesdays and Fridays through professional referral. This is currently a trial service, but it is hoped a more extensive programme of therapies will become available to clients and staff, including Reflexology and Indian Head (& Neck) Massage

Cost: All free of charge

Promotion: Staff refer patients who are anxious or depressed

St John's Hospice in Wirral

Sally Derbyshire, Patient Services Manager   **0151 334 2778**

Mount Road, Higher Bebington, The Wirral, Merseyside CH63 6JE

A specialist palliative care unit serving the Wirral

Therapies: Aromatherapy, Art Therapy, Counselling, Nutritional Supplements

Details: All therapies are available to clients on Tuesday to Friday (09.00-13.00) by professional referral, with Aromatherapy and Counselling open to carers and staff. To be booked in advance

Cost: All free of charge

Quality assurance: Assessment process by professional

Promotion: Leaflets. Posters. On admission to the system. Verbal communication

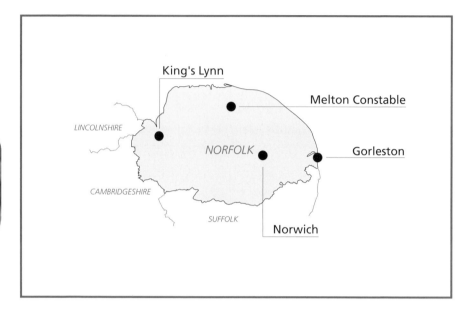

Complementary therapy services in

Norfolk

Gorleston   ● James Paget Healthcare NHS Trust
King's Lynn   ● Tapping House Hospice
Melton Constable   ● Briningham Complementary Cancer Care
Norwich   ● hug - art & crafts for women touched by cancer
                       ● Norfolk & Norwich University NHS Hospital Trust

James Paget Healthcare NHS Trust

Mrs Baxter-Pownall   **01493 452744**
Lowestoft Road, Gorleston, Norfolk NR31 6LA

Although based in an acute setting, the facility provides a seamless service between hospital and community, thereby offering our patients continuity

Therapies:	Acupuncture, Aromatherapy, Massage
Details:	Available to clients on Thursday afternoons by professional referral, with Aromatherapy and Massage available to carers. All therapies require advance booking
Cost:	All free of charge
Quality assurance:	Complementary therapy Steering Group. Policy for use of essential oils. Consent forms. Information leaflets
Materials supplied:	Relaxation tapes
Promotion:	Letters to GPs; posters

Tapping House Hospice

Jan Smith, Macmillan Holistic Care Manager   **01485 543163**
Common Road (West), Snettisham, King's Lynn, Norfolk PE31 7PF

The hospice is an holistic day care centre providing day and home palliative care

Therapies:	Massage, Reflexology, Reiki, Relaxation
Details:	All therapies are available on weekdays, except Thursdays to clients and carers through self referral, although clients can also be referred by health professionals. The facility is currently developing a service which will provide creative therapies
Cost:	All free of charge
Quality assurance:	All patients are assessed by a specialist nurse before any care or therapy is given. GP/consultant advised that complementary

therapies have been requested and asked to contact us if any complementary therapies are contra-indicated. If there is any uncertainty, medical/nursing specialists are contacted directly. Information available and provided to patients, carers and professionals

Materials supplied: CDs, videos, cassettes, books, leaflets (eg. Bristol Cancer Help Centre and CancerBACUP material)

Promotion: Information leaflets/brochures/newsletters/articles in local press/presentations; word of mouth

Briningham Complementary Cancer Care

James & P I Howlett, Owners & Organisers   **01263 860274/861555**
Briningham House, Briningham, Melton Constable, Norfolk NR24 2QJ

A large country house and gardens lend themselves ideally as a venue for the two-day seminars run four times a year

Therapies: Aromatherapy, Dance Therapy, Herbal Remedies, Homeopathy, Massage, Meditation, Music Therapy, Naturopathy, Nutritional Programmes, Reflexology, Relaxation, Spiritual Healing, Nutritional Supplements, Therapeutic Touch, Visualisation

Details: All therapies are available to clients and carers on Fridays and Saturdays through self referral, with Meditation, Naturopathy, Nutritional Programmes, Relaxation, Nutritional Supplements and Visualisation also open to staff. Advance booking is required

Cost: Fees charged

Quality assurance: No – patients can choose complementary therapies appropriate to them

Materials supplied: Cassettes, books on nutrition and on all aspects of cancer healing, visualisation, etc

Promotion: Brochures and leaflet inserts; website; hospitals, consultant surgeons and GP surgeries; Macmillan/breast care nurses; voluntary cancer care groups

hug – art & crafts for women touched by cancer

Rita Evans or Janet Marshall   **01603 411343/438134**
9 Church Green, Norwich, Norfolk NR7 8BA

The local 'Big C' cancer charity has freely allowed the use of space above its premises

Therapies:	Art Therapy
Details:	Available on Friday afternoons to clients on a self referral, drop-in basis
Cost:	All free of charge
Quality assurance:	No – patients choose their own activity
Materials supplied:	Information about other local groups and cancer group link; Macmillan leaflets, Cancerlink directory etc
Promotion:	Leaflets in the Norfolk & Norwich Hospital, Cancer Information Centre and any other suitable sites, eg., Women's Health Centre

Norfolk & Norwich University NHS Hospital Trust

Gill Pout, Haematology Nurse Specialist   **01603 286286 bleep 579**
Brunswick Road, Norwich, Norfolk NR1 3SR

Therapies:	Aromatherapy, Massage
Details:	Available to clients and carers on Monday mornings, Tuesday mornings and Thursday mornings through self referral. Advance booking is required
Cost:	All free of charge
Promotion:	Leaflets and poster on day unit and wards

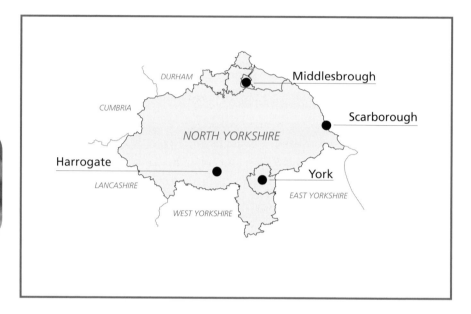

Complementary therapy services in

North Yorkshire

Harrogate	● Yorkshire Cancer Help Centre
Middlesbrough	● Holistic Cancer Care Project
	● James Cook University Hospital
	● South Tees Hospitals NHS Trust
	● Teesside Hospice
Scarborough	● St Catherine's Hospice
York	● Cancer Concern
	● York District Hospital

Yorkshire Cancer Help Centre

Esme Paterson or Ann Scott **Esme – 01423 881392**
or Ann – 0113 216 8894

3 Station View, Harrogate, North Yorkshire HG2 7JA

From a suite of rooms in the parish centre of a church, full and half-day programmes are run to include counselling, healing, relaxation/visualisation and a range of complementary therapies. On full days, an organic, vegetarian lunch is provided

Therapies:	Aromatherapy, Counselling, Massage, Nutritional Programmes, Reflexology, Reiki, Relaxation, Spiritual Healing, Visualisation
Details:	Available to clients and carers through self referral on two Saturdays a month in the mornings and afternoons, with Aromatherapy, Massage, Nutritional Programmes, Reflexology, Reiki, Relaxation, Spiritual Healing and Visualisation open to staff. All therapies operated on a drop-in basis
Cost:	All free of charge
Quality assurance:	Patients and carers are offered 30-45 minute samplers of a range of complementary therapies during the course of the day. Unable to offer series of treatments. If patients feel benefit from specific complementary therapy, they are encouraged to locate someone in their own area. Our therapists are very sensitive to each patient's condition
Materials supplied:	Information pack which includes a page on each complementary therapy offered; books and tapes to buy or borrow
Promotion:	Leaflets and posters; occasional newspaper advertisements and editorials; occasional radio promotions; open days; referrals from nurses

Holistic Cancer Care Project

Sue Stephenson, Manager – Complementary Therapies   01642 854839

c/o The James Cook University Hospital, Marton Road, Middlesbrough, North
Yorkshire TS4 3BW

Funded by donations, this purpose-built, holistic cancer care centre (including an
information centre) should be finished by April 2002. It will be a peaceful place where
oncology/radiotherapy patients, and their carers, can access complementary therapies
free of charge

Therapies:	Acupuncture, Aromatherapy, Counselling, Reflexology, Reiki, Relaxation, Visualisation
Details:	All therapies are available to clients and carers on Monday mornings, Tuesday afternoons, Wednesdays (including evening), Thursdays and Fridays through self referral. Acupuncture, Aromatherapy, Counselling, Reflexology, Relaxation and Visualisation are also available to staff. Advance booking is required
Cost:	All free of charge
Quality assurance:	Information leaflet given to patients. Policies/protocols in place. Developing guidelines for aromatherapists working with the patient with cancer
Materials supplied:	Small selection of literature, books, videos and audio cassettes
Promotion:	Leaflets; posters in department; display in department; through primary care radiographers; through giving talks to local community groups, health professionals and peripheral hospitals

James Cook University Hospital

Dr J E Chandler, Consultant Haematologist　　　　**01642 850850 x5696**
Ward 33, Middlesbrough General Hospital, Ayresome Green Lane, Middlesbrough,
North Yorkshire TS5 5AZ

Therapies:	Aromatherapy, Massage, Reflexology, Relaxation
Details:	All therapies are offered to clients and carers on Tuesday mornings and Thursday mornings on professional referral, with Aromatherapy, Massage and Reflexology open to staff
Cost:	Please enquire
Quality assurance:	Qualified aromatherapist assesses patient/carer before any treatment is given. Any queries are discussed with the consultant
Materials supplied:	Cassettes, vidoes, television
Promotion:	Leaflets and posters

South Tees Hospitals NHS Trust

Andrea Harris, Staff Nurse　　　　**01642 854503**
c/o Ward 3, James Cook University Hospital, Marton Road, Middlesbrough, North
Yorkshire TS4 3BW

An inpatient unit for oncology and haematology patients, also offering day units for
chemotherapy and haematology

Therapies:	Aromatherapy, Massage, Reflexology, Reiki, Relaxation, Visualisation
Details:	Available to clients and carers on Tuesday and Thursday mornings, and Sunday evenings, with Aromatherapy, Massage, Reflexology, Reiki and Relaxation open to staff Massage, Reiki, Relaxation and Visualisation are available through self referral or can be referred by a healthcare professional. Advance booking is required
Cost:	Please enquire

Quality assurance:	Protocol consists of providing information leaflets and assessment by a complementary practitioner
Materials supplied:	Information leaflets
Promotion:	Posters and leaflets; radio interview

Teesside Hospice

01642 816777

1a Northgate Road, Linthorpe, Middlesbrough, North Yorkshire TS5 5NW

Hospice day care taking up to 16 guests per day Monday to Thursday

Therapies:	Aromatherapy, Art Therapy, Massage, Music Therapy, Reflexology, Reiki, Relaxation, Spiritual Healing, Visualisation
Details:	Therapies are available to clients on Mondays, Tuesdays, Wednesday afternoons, Thursday afternoons and Friday afternoons, with Aromatherapy open to carers and staff. All are on self referral except Relaxation and Visualisation
Cost:	Free of charge for Aromatherapy, Art Therapy, Massage, Reflexology, Spiritual Healing There is a fee for Music Therapy
Quality assurance:	Aromatherapy protocol in place. Aromatherapist assessment procedure. Referral system
Promotion:	Verbally through attendance at day care; information booklet for patients

St Catherine's Hospice

Jackie Bolton   **01723 351421**

137 Scalby Road, Scarborough, North Yorkshire YO12 6TB

St Catherine's Hospice is a charitable organisation providing specialist palliative care

Therapies:	Acupuncture, Aromatherapy, Neuro-Linguistic Programming

Details: Available to clients on professional referral (contact for details of availability). Advance booking is required
Cost: All free of charge
Quality assurance: Assessment by referring professional and the therapist providing the service
Materials supplied: Leaflets
Promotion: Promote to health professionals, eg. GPs, Macmillan and district nurses

Cancer Concern

Mitzi Blennerhassett, Co-ordinator　　　　　　　**01653 628369**
Wyville Lodge, Slingsby, York, North Yorkshire

A self-help and support group which meets monthly in York. Therapists attend, but in the main treat in their own homes, and sometimes in clients' homes

Therapies: Acupuncture, Aromatherapy, Counselling, Hypnotherapy/Hypnosis, Massage, Relaxation, Visualisation
Details: Available to clients and carers on self referral. Availability of therapies varies to fit in with clients' needs and when therapists are available (contact for details of availability). Advance booking for Acupuncture, Aromatherapy, Counselling and Massage (clients can be referred for Aromatherapy and Massage by healthcare professional); Relaxation available on drop-in
Cost: All free of charge
Quality assurance: Patients advised to inform GP or consultant before undertaking therapies. Therapists fully qualified and experienced in dealing with cancer
Materials supplied: Literature available at meetings; clients may also ring therapists for discussion on subject
Promotion: Leaflets; hospital waiting rooms; GPs' surgeries; occasional press coverage

York District Hospital

Dr Anne Garry, Consultant in Palliative Medicine   **01904 725830**
Wigginton Road, York, North Yorkshire YO31 8HE

Therapies:	Aromatherapy, Art Therapy, Massage, Reflexology
Details:	Available to clients on Monday afternoons, Wednesdays and Fridays by self referral (Art Therapy) and professional referral (all therapies). Advance booking for for Aromatherapy, Massage and Reflexology
Cost:	All free of charge
Quality assurance:	All touch therapists have a health/cancer care background
Promotion:	Leaflets at cancer care centre in York District Hospital and with healthcare professionals

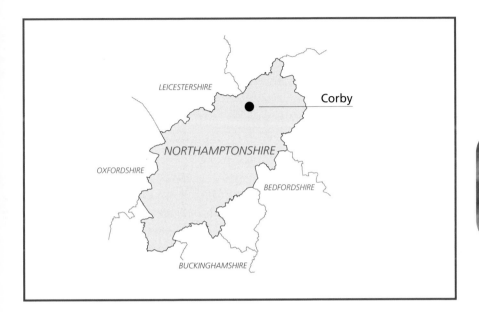

Complementary therapy services in

Northamptonshire

Corby   ● Lakelands Hospice

Lakelands Hospice

Ella Fullerton, Hospice Manager   **01536 747755**

Butland Road, Oakley Vale, Corby, Northamptonshire NN18 8LX

Provision of day care

Therapies:	Aromatherapy, Art Therapy, Massage, Music Therapy, Nutritional Programmes, Reflexology, Reiki, Relaxation, Nutritional Supplements, Therapeutic Touch
Details:	Available to clients on Tuesdays, Wednesdays (including evenings) and Thursdays by self referral. Aromatherapy, Art Therapy, Massage, Music Therapy, Reflexology and Relaxation are available to carers and staff
	Patients can be referred by health professionals for Nutritional Supplements and Nutritional Programmes
Cost:	Please enquire
Quality assurance:	Medical evidence. Diagnosis of patient. History of patient
Materials supplied:	Brochure
Promotion:	Brochure; posters; media/radio/tv/newspaper; GPs' surgeries

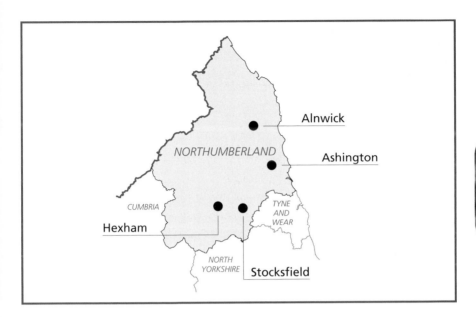

Complementary therapy services in

Northumberland

Alnwick	• North Northumberland Day Hospice
	• Northumbria Healthcare NHS Trust
Ashington	• Central Palz
Hexham	• Northumbria Healthcare NHS Trust
Stocksfield	• Northumberland Cancer Support Group

North Northumberland Day Hospice

Joan Robson, Day Hospice Sister　　　　　　　　　**01665 606515**
Castleside House, 40 Narrowgate, Alnwick, Northumberland NE66 1JQ

Day hospice care led by nurses at two sites, Alnwick and Berwick, is integrated with community services

Therapies:	Aromatherapy, Art Therapy, Massage, Music Therapy, Reflexology, Relaxation
Details:	All therapies are available to clients on Tuesdays, Wednesday afternoons and Thursdays, with Aromatherapy, Massage, Reflexology and Relaxation open to carers. All patients are referred via healthcare professionals, but carers can self-refer
Cost:	All free of charge
Quality assurance:	Standards in place. GP must return signed consent form prior to treatment. Staff nurse with complementary therapy training holds supervised sessions with volunteer therapists
Promotion:	Leaflets; discussions with individuals

Northumbria Healthcare NHS Trust

Sister C Gattens　　　　　　　　　**01665 626753**
Aln Ward, Alnwick Infirmary, Alnwick, Northumberland NE65 8DZ

A GP-run community hospital

Therapies:	Acupuncture, Aromatherapy, Massage, Relaxation
Details:	All therapies available to clients (contact for details of availability) with Relaxation open to staff. Aromatherapy, Massage, Relaxation are on self referral
Cost:	All free of charge
Quality assurance:	Patients self-refer, but referral must be approved by medical staff. All staff have basic training in relaxation and in massaging hands and feet. All staff know which treatments are appropriate
Promotion:	Noticeboard on the ward; word of mouth

Central Palz

Liz Harmer, Lead Nurse   **01670 842021**

c/o Seaton Hirst Primary Care Centre, Norham Road, Ashington, Northumberland
NE63 0NG

Central Palz runs every Wednesday and Thursday providing a service for patients and
carers with palliative needs. The group is situated in a local GP practice providing a
service to the whole of central Northumberland

Therapies:	Aromatherapy, Counselling, Massage, Reflexology
Details:	Available to clients and carers on Wednesdays and Thursdays through professional referral
Cost:	All free of charge
Quality assurance:	Information leaflets. Tailor-made treatments for each individual. Evidence-based practice
Materials supplied:	Booklets, internet access, information from nurse specialists, videos
Promotion:	Central Palz leaflet; quarterly newsletter; information leaflets for patients/carers; regular newspaper articles

Northumbria Healthcare NHS Trust

E Bowden, Macmillan Nurse   **01434 604008**

Hexham General Hospital, Community Offices, Corbridge Road, Hexham,
Northumberland NE46 1QJ

The trust works in the community, but also crosses boundaries into hospitals and
nursing homes in the area. It is also heavily involved with Tynedale community
hospice, which takes care into patients' homes

Therapies:	Aromatherapy, Counselling, Massage, Reflexology, Relaxation
Details:	Available to clients and carers on weekdays including evenings through professional referral
Cost:	Please enquire

Quality assurance:	Cross-check with referrers: district/Macmillan nurse or GP/oncologist or palliative consultant
Materials supplied:	Written material, leaflets about other complementary therapists in the area and their costs
Promotion:	Leaflets, but mostly by word of mouth through Macmillan and district nurses. Tynedale Community Hospice advertises its services, which includes this partnership. Also aware of other organisations in area offering complementary therapies and give out information on when/where/cost

Northumberland Cancer Support Group

Linda Brinkhurst, Secretary   **01661 842919**

c/o 47 Apperley Road, Stocksfield, Northumberland NE43 7PQ

Therapies:	Alexander Technique, Aromatherapy, Counselling, Massage, Indian Head (& Neck) Massage, Reflexology, Reiki, Shiatsu, Nutritional Supplements
Available:	Available to clients and carers on Tuesday evenings through self referral. Therapies vary on availability of volunteers (this list represents the current position). Can only offer up to four therapies at any one meeting. Therapies available to volunteers
Cost:	Free of charge for Alexander Technique, Aromatherapy, Counselling, Massage, Indian Head (& Neck) Massage, Reflexology, Reiki, Shiatsu
There is a fee for Nutritional Supplements.
Quality assurance:	Volunteer therapists work within strict guidelines and code of practice. Written guidelines approved by local lead clinician for cancer services. Therapists take patient's history before treatment
Materials supplied:	Library of books, tapes, etc. NCSG information pack; Bristol Cancer Help centre video and information pack
Promotion:	Posters; leaflets; cards; newspaper advertisement

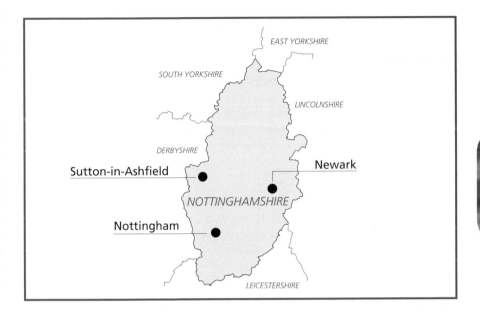

Complementary therapy services in

Nottinghamshire

Newark	● Beaumond House Community Hospice
Nottingham	● Nottingham Cancer Patients Support Group
	● Nottingham City Hospital NHS Trust
	● Queens Medical Centre
	● The Nottinghamshire Hospice
Sutton-in-Ashfield	● John Eastwood Hospice

Beaumond House Community Hospice

Christine Smith, Assistant Care Manager   **01636 610556**

32 London Road, Newark, Nottinghamshire NG24 1TW

Therapies:	Aromatherapy, Massage
Details:	All therapies are available to clients, carers and staff on Tuesdays, Thursdays and Friday afternoons by self referral. Book in advance for all therapies
Cost:	All free of charge
Quality assurance:	Masseurs are appropriately qualified. Liaison with patient's GP/consultant. Liaison with patient's Macmillan nurse
Promotion:	In brochure; by word of mouth

Nottingham Cancer Patients Support Group

Freda E Ingall RGN   **0115 9313541**

Beckside, 1 Grange Close, Lambley, Nottingham, Nottinghamshire NG4 4QJ

A voluntary group holding monthly meetings at Queen's Medical Centre, Nottingham and running craft days and social activities at other venues. It supports local HAZ roadshows. In contact with trainee healthcare professionals and postgraduate educators

Therapies:	Relaxation, Therapeutic Touch, Visualisation
Details:	Available to clients, carers and staff through monthly meetings on Tuesday evenings (available at other times by discussion with the service provider). All therapies are available on self referral. Relaxation and Visualisation are on a drop-in basis. Regular speakers talk on Meditation, Reiki, Herbal Remedies, Nutritional Supplements, Nutritional Programmes, Aromatherapy, Massage, Reflexology, Shiatsu, Osteopathy and Chiropractic therapies

Cost:	All free of charge
Materials supplied:	Library of books, videos and tapes covering most complementary therapies; also have Bristol Cancer Help Centre's videos and tapes
Promotion:	Leaflets; announcements at meetings; radio announcements; local newspaper; phone members and send out invitations

Nottingham City Hospital NHS Trust

Ms June Mew, Complementary Therapy Practitioner   **0115 9627619**
CT Unit, Hayward House Macmillan Specialist Palliative Care, Hucknall Road, Nottingham, Nottinghamshire NG5 1PB

The complementary therapy unit is a purpose-built extension in pine offering four individual therapy rooms, each furnished with comfortable chairs and a couch. A quiet environment supports the aim of promoting relaxation from the therapies offered

Therapies:	Acupuncture, Aromatherapy, Massage, Reflexology, Relaxation, Visualisation
Details:	Available to clients on weekdays through professional referral, with Aromatherapy, Massage and Reflexology open to staff. Advance booking required
Cost:	All free of charge
Quality assurance:	Information is given when initial discussion on complementary therapies takes place with practitioner. Tailored to individual's needs and condition
Materials supplied:	Leaflets on therapies available
Promotion:	Leaflets on the therapies available; via Macmillan nurses, day care and inpatient staff

Queens Medical Centre

Virginia McGivern, Senior Staff Nurse **0115 924 9924**
Nottingham University Hospital, Ward E38, Children's Day Care, Derby Road,
Nottingham, Nottinghamshire NG7 2UH

Queens Medical Centre provides an oncology/medical ward for children

Therapies:	Aromatherapy, Counselling, Massage, Relaxation, Therapeutic Touch, Visualisation
Details:	Therapies available to clients and carers on Friday afternoons and evenings, with Aromatherapy, Counselling, Massage, Relaxation and Therapeutic Touch open to staff. All therapies except Counselling are available through self referral or can either be referred by a healthcare professional, or booked on drop-in
Cost:	All free of charge. One day a year a session is held for staff and a nominal fee is charged, not full rates
Quality assurance:	Medication – contra-indications need to be noted on referral form. Consultation takes between 10 and 30 minutes. Discussion with nursing/medical staff. Reading of medical notes
Materials supplied:	Books/magazines always available; safety information on essential oils used
Promotion:	Word of mouth; information leaflet in the oncology file and on the notice board

The Nottinghamshire Hospice

Julie Tovey, Palliative Care Services Manager **0115 910 1008**
'Fernleigh', 384 Woodborough Road, Nottingham, Nottinghamshire NG3 4JF

A community-based hospice providing day care and nursing at home

Therapies:	Aromatherapy, Art Therapy, Massage, Meditation, Music Therapy, Reflexology, Relaxation, Shiatsu, Spiritual Healing, Yoga

Details:	All therapies are available to clients on weekdays through professional referral. Aromatherapy, Massage, Meditation, Reflexology, Relaxation, Shiatsu and Spiritual Healing therapies are open to carers, with Yoga available to staff
Cost:	Free of charge for Aromatherapy, Art Therapy, Massage, Music Therapy, Reflexology, Relaxation, Shiatsu, Spiritual Healing. A fee is charged for Yoga
Quality assurance:	All patients are referred to the hospice by a GP or district nurse. All day care patients are offered complementary therapies, but GP must sign to agree individual therapies (checks for contra-indications, etc.)
Promotion:	In-house service (part of regular provision); leaflets on services; letters to GPs and district nurses

John Eastwood Hospice

Helen Dowell, Complementary Therapy Co-ordinator   **01623 622626 x281**
Mansfield Road, Sutton-in-Ashfield, Nottinghamshire NG17 4HJ

Therapies:	Acupuncture, Aromatherapy, Massage, Reflexology, Reiki
Details:	All therapies are available to clients on all weekdays except Thursday afternoon through professional referral, with Aromatherapy and Massage open to carers and staff, and Reflexology and Reiki additionally open to carers. Advance booking required
Cost:	All free of charge
Quality assurance:	A complementary therapist assesses patient at first meeting before proceeding with treatment. Medical notes of inpatient or day care patients available for information on their condition. Diagnosis and reasons for referral are included on referral form
Promotion:	Leaflets in day care files for Aromatherapy, Reflexology and Reiki, but not for home use; verbal communication through staff/Macmillan nurses and rest of multidisciplinary team; verbal communication with complementary therapist; currently developing Aromatherapy leaflet to give clients and carers

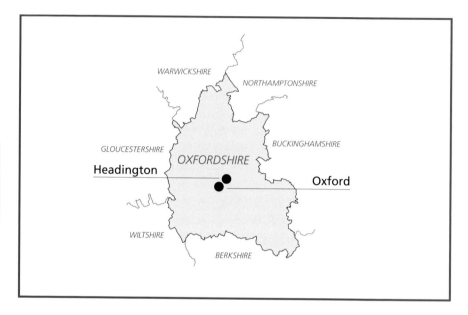

Complementary therapy services in

Oxfordshire

Headington
Oxford

- Abernethy Cancer Information Centre
- John Radcliffe Hospital
- Sir Michael Sobell House

Abernethy Cancer Information Centre

Helen Elphick   **01865 225690**

Oxford Radcliffe Trust, The Churchill Hospital, Old Road, Headington, Oxfordshire
OX3 7LJ

Therapies:	Aromatherapy, Art Therapy, Counselling, Massage, Reflexology, Relaxation, Spiritual Healing
Details:	Available to clients on weekdays through self referral (some holistic workshops run on an occasional basis on Saturdays). Diet workshops run by NHS staff
Cost:	All free of charge
Quality assurance:	A set of guidelines is available in line with requirement of Trust's executive board. Guidelines outline the operational policy and safe practice protocol
Promotion:	Leaflets; posters; displays; talks to health professionals, students, Oxford Cancer Services Advisory Group

John Radcliffe Hospital

The Palliative Care Support Team   **01865 221741**

c/o Corridor 6C/D, Palliative Care Support Team, Headington, Oxford, Oxfordshire
OX3 9DU

Therapies:	Acupuncture, Aromatherapy, Art Therapy, Massage, Music Therapy, Reflexology
Details:	Available to clients in response to need, subject to availability through professional referral (the palliative care support team does not have complementary therapies integral to its service but these are available through the Michael Sobell Hospice)
Cost:	Please enquire
Quality assurance:	First discussed with lead consultant in charge of patient's care at hospital. Complementary therapy co-ordinator aware of contra-indications for complementary therapies. Any referral would involve taking relevant medical history
Promotion:	Through consultation with clients and staff education

Sir Michael Sobell House

Nigel Hartley, Complementary Therapy Co-ordinator   **01865 225371**
Churchill Hospital, Old Road, Headington, Oxford, Oxfordshire OX3 7LJ

The facility includes a 20-bed inpatient unit, a day centre for up to 15 people a week, bereavement, outpatient and complementary therapy services

Therapies:	Acupuncture, Aromatherapy, Art Therapy, Massage, Music Therapy, Reflexology, Relaxation
Details:	Available to clients, carers and staff on Mondays (including evenings), Tuesdays (including evenings), Wednesday mornings and evenings, Thursday mornings and evenings, Fridays and Saturday evenings through self referral (can also be referred by a healthcare professional). Advance booking required for all therapies
Cost:	All free of charge
Quality assurance:	Therapist links with patient's key nurse. With patient's permission, therapist takes history at first session
Promotion:	Information leaflet

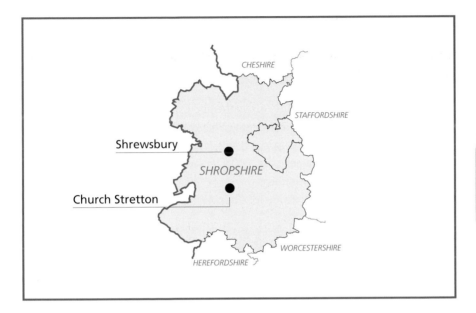

Complementary therapy services in

Shropshire

Church Stretton	• Stretton Cancer Care
Shrewsbury	• Hamar Help & Support Centre
	• Shropshire & Mid-Wales Hospice

Stretton Cancer Care

Robin Jukes-Hughes, Co-ordinator   **01694 724024**
The Cottage, Cwmdale, Church Stretton, Shropshire SY6 6JL

Therapies:	Acupuncture, Aromatherapy, Counselling, Homeopathy, Massage, Osteopathy, Reflexology, Shiatsu, Spiritual Healing, Nutritional Supplements, Visualisation
Details:	All therapies are available to clients through self referral and by appointment
Cost:	Free of charge for Counselling, Nutritional Supplements, Visualisation
	There is a fee for Acupuncture, Aromatherapy, Homeopathy, Massage, Osteopathy, Reflexology, Shiatsu, Spiritual Healing
Quality assurance:	Guidance is provided on choice of therapies if requested
Materials supplied:	A wide range of books, pamphlets, videos and cassettes is available

Hamar Help & Support Centre

Wendy Thompson RGN, BSc (Hons), MA, Team Leader   **01743 261035**
Royal Shrewsbury Hospital North, Mytton Oak Road, Shrewsbury, Shropshire SY3 8XQ

Occupying a purpose-built unit on the hospital site and originally funded by a local oncology charity, the Support Centre is now funded by the hospital. It maintains close links with the local community and hospice

Therapies:	Aromatherapy, Art Therapy, Counselling, Reiki, Relaxation, Therapeutic Touch
Details:	Available to clients and carers. Counselling is available on all weekdays; Therapeutic Touch and Reiki are available on Tuesdays; Aromatherapy on Thursdays; Art Therapy on Wednesday mornings and Relaxation on Wednesday afternoons. Professional referral is required for Aromatherapy, Art Therapy, Reiki, Relaxation and Therapeutic Touch; self referrals accepted for Counselling

Cost:	All free of charge
Quality assurance:	All clients, who can self-refer, have to meet with either the Centre's team leader or a nurse/counsellor. They discuss options of support/therapies with general assessment of their situation and needs. Account is taken of clients' psychological/emotional state, condition and treatments' side effects. In discussion with the client, an assessment is made of which approach would be the most helpful
Materials supplied:	Individual sheets for each approach
Promotion:	Leaflets; posters and flyers; information packs given out by specialist nurses and at oncology clinics

Shropshire & Mid-Wales Hospice

Annette Rushton, Matron   **01743 261519/236565**
Bicton Heath, Shrewsbury, Shropshire SY3 8HS

Therapies:	Acupuncture, Aromatherapy, Art Therapy, Counselling, Music, Reflexology
Details:	Available to clients on weekdays through professional referral
Cost:	Free of charge for Aromatherapy, Art Therapy, Counselling, Music Therapy, Reflexology There is a fee for Acupuncture
Quality assurance:	All patients are reviewed by a doctor prior to being referred on for therapy. Therapists liaise very closely with the medical and nursing teams. Policies are in place to ensure good practice
Promotion:	These therapies are offered to patients attending the day hospice or admitted to the day unit

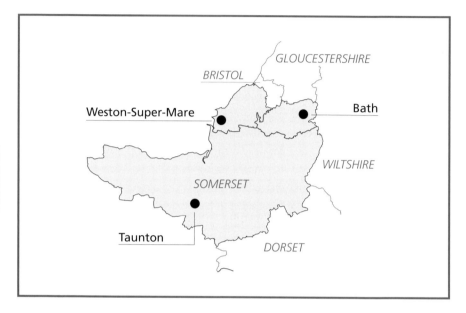

Complementary therapy services in

Somerset

Bath	● Royal United Hospital NHS Trust
Taunton	● Somerset Cancer Care
	● St Margaret's Somerset Hospice
	● Taunton & Somerset Hospital
Weston-Super-Mare	● Weston Area Health Trust

Royal United Hospital NHS Trust

Hilary Taylor   **01225 825097**

Oncology Directorate, Combe Park, Bath, Somerset BA1 3NG

The Trust's oncology directorate provides chemotherapy, radiotherapy and symptom management to oncology and haematology patients over the age of 16

Therapies:	Aromatherapy, Massage, Reflexology
Details:	Available to clients and carers on Tuesday mornings and evenings through self referral. Advance booking is required
Cost:	All free of charge
	Massage and Reflexology are also available at alternative times for a fee
Quality assurance:	Guidelines specified. Consultant aware of treatment being offered. No Massage to tumour site. Platelet count over 50 before Massage applied
Promotion:	Posters; staff recommend service

Somerset Cancer Care

Christine Canti for patients and carers   **01823 421623/432450**
                                                                                       for health professionals

Sandhill Park House, Ash Priors, Taunton, Somerset TA4 3NG

Complementary therapies are provided for patients and carers at three area support groups (Minehead, Taunton and Mendip). Some therapies can be offered to patients at the local hospital's outpatient chemotherapy and oncology clinics

Therapies:	Aromatherapy, Massage, Reflexology, Reiki, Relaxation, Spiritual Healing, Visualisation
Details:	Available to clients and staff on self referral on drop in. The Minehead group operates on Monday afternoons; the Taunton

group on Thursday evenings; the Mendip group on Friday afternoons. There is a monthly session on Wednesday evenings for chemotherapy patients at Taunton Hospital. Hand massage is offered at oncology clinics Monday to Thursday. Volunteers are trained in counselling/listening skills, but an agreed period of one-to-one counselling is not provided. Aromatherapy and Reflexology not always available

Cost: All free of charge

Quality assurance: Aromatherapists, reflexologists and healers are all trained and the groups work closely with cancer professionals at their local hospital

Promotion: Leaflets; posters; word of mouth; press

St Margaret's Somerset Hospice

Mrs Jean Thomas   **01823 259394**
Heron Drive, Bishops Hull, Taunton, Somerset TA1 5HA

St Margaret's provides a 16-bed inpatient unit, a day care service, a community nursing service and a hospital liaison team

Therapies: Acupuncture, Aromatherapy, Massage, Reflexology, Relaxation, Visualisation

Details: Therapies available to clients on weekdays through professional referral, with Aromatherapy, Massage and Reflexology open to carers

Cost: All free of charge

Quality assurance: There is a complementary therapy co-ordinator who assesses new referrals. Written guidelines

Materials supplied: Relaxation tapes and literature as appropriate

Promotion: Through day care and inpatient units; through community palliative care nurse specialists

Taunton & Somerset Hospital

Sister Caren Beardon   **01823 342009**

Palliative Care Unit, Ward 9, Musgrove Park, Taunton, Somerset TA1 5DA

A 4-bedded, palliative care unit within a district general hospital

Therapies:	Acupuncture, Aromatherapy, Chiropractic, Counselling, Massage, Nutritional Supplements
Details:	Availability to clients to suit patient and practitioner, with Aromatherapy and Counselling open to carers and staff, and Massage also available to staff. Professional referral required for Acupuncture, Aromatherapy, Chiropractic and Massage; self referral accepted for Counselling and Nutritional Supplements. All therapies except Nutritional Supplements require advance booking
Cost:	All free of charge
Quality assurance:	Given by trained therapist after consultation with nurse
Promotion:	Leaflets; posters; word of mouth

Weston Area Health Trust

Corrine Thomas, Clinical Nurse Specialist Oncology   01934 636363 x3652/3653
Oncology Unit, Grange Road, Uphill, Weston-Super-Mare, Somerset BS23 4TQ

The Trust oncology day unit caters for outpatients; although small, it is expected to expand in 2002

Therapies:	Aromatherapy, Massage, Reflexology
Details:	Aromatherapy and Massage (including hand massage) are available to clients and staff on Monday mornings and Tuesday mornings on professional referral. Additionally, Reflexology is available to staff. Advance booking is required

Cost:	Charges apply for staff
Quality assurance:	Local hospice and Bristol oncology centre is aware of appropriate treatment
Materials supplied:	Leaflets and videos; there are plans to include a resource room in the extension
Promotion:	Verbally tell patients about Hand Massage offered at the unit; verbally tell and have booklets for patients about Aromatherapy offered at local hospice; verbally tell and leaflets for patients regarding 'Look Good Feel Good' session at Bristol Oncology Centre. Complementary therapies to commence for a fee in the Trust for staff from January 2002

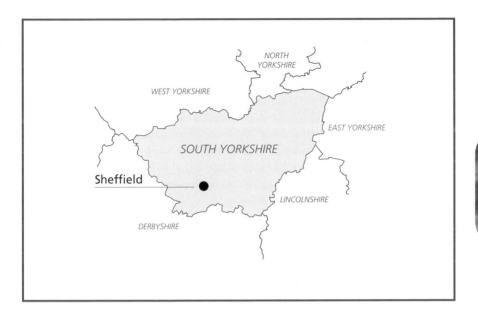

Complementary therapy services in

South Yorkshire

Sheffield
- St Luke's Hospice
- The Cavendish Centre for Cancer Care
- Weston Park Hospital

St Luke's Hospice

Margaret Carradice, Matron   **0114 236 2271**
Little Common Lane, off Abbey Lane, Sheffield, South Yorkshire S11 9NE

Therapies:	Acupuncture, Aromatherapy, Art Therapy, Massage, Reflexology, Relaxation, Shiatsu, Nutritional Supplements
Details:	All therapies are available to clients on weekdays through self referral, with Acupuncture and Shiatsu open to staff. Clients can be referred for complementary therapies by health professionals
Cost:	All free of charge
Promotion:	Leaflets; personal approach by therapists

The Cavendish Centre for Cancer Care

Dr Andrew Manasse   **0114 278 4600**
27 Wilkinson Street, Sheffield, South Yorkshire S10 2GB

Based on the ground floor of a Regency house close to, but separate from, the local oncology hospital and the major hospital trust

Therapies:	Acupuncture, Aromatherapy, Art Therapy, Counselling, Homeopathy, Massage, Meditation, Reflexology, Reiki, Relaxation, Shiatsu, Spiritual Healing, Visualisation
Details:	All therapies are available to clients and carers on weekdays including Thursday evenings through self referral. Acupuncture, Aromatherapy, Homeopathy, Massage, Reflexology, Reiki, Shiatsu and Spiritual Healing therapies are available to staff Book in advance for all therapies. Each patient has an hour-long assessment during which an appropriate choice of therapy is negotiated

Cost:	Please enquire
Materials supplied:	There is a small library of selected books and leaflets
Promotion:	Posters and leaflets in hospital departments and GP surgeries; direct communication with hospital and community nurses; volunteer speakers eg., addressing women's groups; staff lecture to allied health professionals and to medical students

Weston Park Hospital

Vicky Gaughan or Sue Roebuck   **0114 226 5000 x5666**
Witham Road, Sheffield, South Yorkshire S10 2SJ

The hospital is a regional cancer care centre offering, among other things, Massage at the patient's bedside

Therapies:	Acupuncture, Massage, Relaxation, Visualisation
Details:	Available to clients on Wednesdays and Thursdays with an Acupuncture clinic available on Friday afternoon. Massage, Relaxation and Visualisation are available through self referral or can be referred by a healthcare professional
Cost:	All free of charge
Quality assurance:	Information leaflet. Care standards. Collection of medical history from discussion with patient and relevant staff
Promotion:	Leaflets; in-house posters

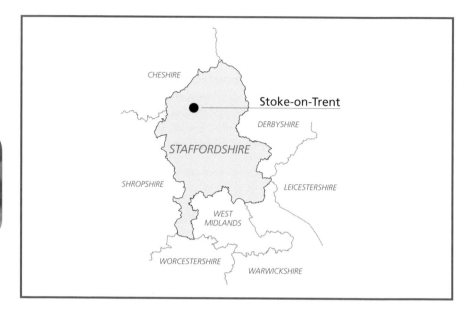

Complementary therapy services in
Staffordshire

Stoke-on-Trent   • The Donna Louise Trust

The Donna Louise Trust

Margaret Harvey, Head of Care   **01782 811911**

95A The Strand, Longton, Stoke-on-Trent, Staffordshire ST3 2NS

Part of an organisation building a children's hospice that is due to open in Summer 2002. A children's community team is in place and will shortly start to work with families

Therapies:	Aromatherapy, Art Therapy, Counselling, Drama Therapy, Music Therapy, Relaxation
Details:	All therapies will be available to clients, carers and staff on self referral
Cost:	All free of charge

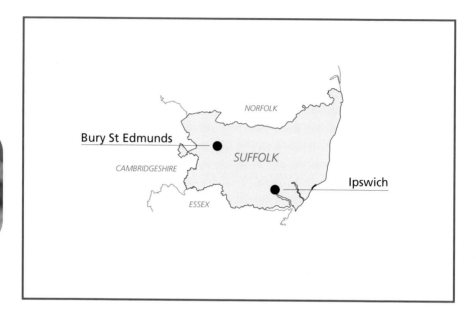

Complementary therapy services in

Suffolk

Bury St Edmunds   • St Nicholas' Hospice
Ipswich   • St Elizabeth Hospice
                        • Suffolk Oncology Centre

St Nicholas' Hospice

Jennifer Field, Clinical Services Manager   **01284 766133**
Macmillan Way, Hardwick Lane, Bury St Edmunds, Suffolk IP33 2QY

Therapies:	Acupuncture, Aromatherapy, Counselling, Massage, Reflexology, Relaxation
Details:	All therapies are available to clients on weekdays except Tuesdays, with Aromatherapy, Counselling, Massage and Reflexology open to carers and staff. Professional referral required for all except Counselling which can be self referred. Therapies should be advance booked
Cost:	A small fee is charged to staff for Aromatherapy, Massage and Reflexology
Promotion:	Leaflet; at assessment for day hospice; Macmillan nurses; hospital palliative care team

St Elizabeth Hospice

Angela Smith, Complementary Therapy Team Leader   **01473 727776**
565 Foxhall Road, Ipswich, Suffolk IP3 8LX

Therapies:	Acupuncture, Aromatherapy, Art Therapy, Counselling, Massage, Reflexology, Reiki, Relaxation, Visualisation
Details:	All therapies are available to clients through self referral on weekdays, with Aromatherapy, Counselling, Massage, Reflexology, Reiki available to carers and staff. Relaxation and Visualisation also available to carers. Book in advance for Acupuncture, Aromatherapy, Art Therapy, Counselling, Massage, Reflexology, Reiki, Relaxation. Clients can be referred for all therapies by health professionals
Cost:	All free of charge

Quality assurance:	Assessment by complementary therapy nurse prior to treatment. All therapists are qualified and receive ongoing training. Multidisciplinary notes used to assess physical, psychological and spiritual status
Materials supplied:	Leaflets, booklets
Promotion:	Leaflets; referrals from community, hospital and hospice staff

Suffolk Oncology Centre

Annie Hallett, Complementary Therapy Coordinator   **01473 704903**

Ipswich Hospital, Heath Road, Ipswich, Suffolk IP4 5PD

Therapies:	Aromatherapy, Counselling, Massage, Meditation, Reflexology, Relaxation, Visualisation
Details:	Available to clients and carers on Mondays to Wednesdays through self referral. All must be booked in advance
Cost:	Please enquire
Quality assurance:	Usually self-referral but health professionals also refer. Initial assessment is made by complementary therapy co-ordinator who is also a nurse. Assessment includes evaluation of possible contra-indications and particular needs of patient/carer
Materials supplied:	Relaxation tapes; CD made by complementary therapy co-ordinator; information on use of essential oils at home
Promotion:	Referral from staff including doctor; leaflets; information booklets; posters

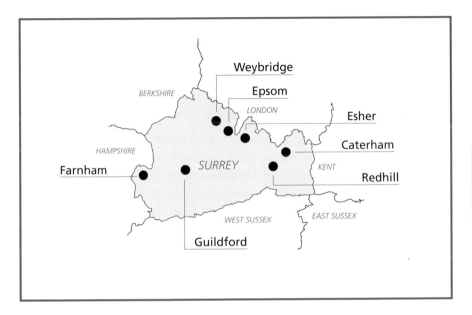

Complementary therapy services in

Surrey

Caterham	● Marie Curie Centre - Caterham
Epsom	● Epsom & St Helier NHS Trust
Esher	● Princess Alice Hospice
Farnham	● Phyllis Tuckwell Hospice
Guildford	● CHASE Children's Hospice Service
	● The Beacon Community Cancer and Palliative Care Centre
	● The Fountain Centre
Redhill	● Surrey & Sussex Healthcare NHS Trust
Weybridge	● Bournewood Community NHS Trust

Marie Curie Cancer Care – Caterham

Mrs Anna Kittel, Occupational Therapist   **01883 832606**
Harestone Drive, Caterham, Surrey CR3 6YQ

A small inpatient unit plus a day therapy unit and a community service

Therapies:	Aromatherapy, Counselling, Hypnotherapy/Hypnosis, Reflexology, Relaxation, Visualisation
Details:	All therapies are available to clients and carers with Counselling open to staff. Open on Wednesday mornings, and Thursday and Friday afternoons on alternate weeks. Also available on Sunday afternoons once a month All therapies require advance booking. Referrals to the centre must be through a doctor. Patients can self-refer once they are clients of the centre
Cost:	Please enquire
Quality assurance:	A form is completed by referring professional or by complementary therapist in conjunction with client either prior to or at first appointment. Form lists cautions/symptoms and allows for documentation of risk limitation action
Materials supplied:	Leaflet
Promotion:	Leaflets; verbal information from staff

Epsom & St Helier NHS Trust

Mrs Wendy Hoy, CT Co-ordinator **01372 735457/735735 bleep 858**
Macmillan Butterfly Centre, Epsom General Hospital, Dorking Road, Epsom, Surrey KT18 7EG

The facility is a new information, drop-in and outpatient centre for cancer patients and their families offering a range of complementary therapies. It also houses many of the outpatient and palliative care clinics, and the relevant staff

Therapies:	Aromatherapy, Counselling, Massage, Meditation, Reflexology, Relaxation, Spiritual Healing, Visualisation

Details: All therapies are available to clients through self referral with Meditation, Relaxation and Visualisation open to carers and staff, and Aromatherapy, Massage and Reflexology additionally available to carers

Open on Mondays to Thursdays, Tuesday evenings and Friday afternoons. Advance booking is available for all therapies with a drop-in service available for Meditation, Relaxation and Visualisation

Cost: All free of charge

Four free sessions are available for Meditation, Relaxation, Visualisation, Aromatherapy, Massage, Reflexology and Spiritual Healing

Quality assurance: Complementary therapy co-ordinator is an oncology/palliative care clinical nurse specialist and qualified aromatherapist. A specific referral form and a clinical assessment form have to be completed. Complementary therapy co-ordinator or CNS may review clients undergoing oncology treatment or who have clinical problems

Materials supplied: Leaflets

Promotion: Via outpatient clinics; leaflets and posters; networking/ drop-in centre; local community advertising

Princess Alice Hospice

Eva Garland, Director of Clinical Services   **01372 461827**
West End Lane, Esher, Surrey KT10 9DL

Provides palliative care to the terminally ill, and help and advice to their families and friends. The team's dedication and expertise has earned its reputation as one of the leaders in the field of caring for the terminally ill

Therapies: Aromatherapy, Art Therapy, Counselling, Massage, Music Therapy, Reflexology, Relaxation

Details:	All therapies are available to clients on weekday afternoons, with Aromatherapy, Art Therapy, Counselling, Massage, Music Therapy and Reflexology open to carers, and Aromatherapy and Counselling open to staff
	Self referrals are accepted for Art Therapy and Music Therapy; professional referrals required for Aromatherapy, Counselling, Massage, Reflexology and Relaxation. (Patients can request, but referral goes through a health professional). There is a Counselling service for the bereaved
Cost:	All free of charge
Promotion:	Leaflets; posters; word of mouth

Phyllis Tuckwell Hospice

Mrs Bridget Purser   **01252 729400**
Waverley Lane, Farnham, Surrey GU9 8BL

A 21-bedded, specialist palliative care hospice caring not only for patients with cancer, but also those with HIV, AIDS, and others suffering from distressing, uncontrolled symptoms

Therapies:	Aromatherapy, Counselling, Massage, Reflexology, Relaxation, Spiritual Healing
Details:	All therapies are available to clients on weekdays plus Friday evenings and Saturday mornings, with Aromatherapy, Counselling, Massage and Reflexology therapies open to carers and staff
	Professional referral is required for Aromatherapy, Counselling, Massage, Reflexology and Spiritual Healing; self referrals are accepted for Counselling and Relaxation. All therapies should be booked in advance
Cost:	All free of charge

Quality assurance: Diagnosis of patient and contra-indications to therapy. Care plan referral form. Referral by therapies co-ordinator or senior medical staff

Materials supplied: Appropriate essential oils for use at home; relaxation tapes/CDs and relaxation exercise sheet

Promotion: Word of mouth by nursing/medical staff; in our hospice brochure/leaflets; wall posters; circulars to carers

CHASE Children's Hospice Service

Chris Robinson, Chief Executive 01483 454213
Loseley Park, Guildford, Surrey GU3 1HS

A children's hospice

Therapies: Aromatherapy, Massage, Music Therapy

Available: Available to clients and carers on weekdays and weekday evenings. Complementary therapies can be arranged when visiting the hospice

Cost: All free of charge

Promotion: In discussion with individual children and their families

The Beacon Community Cancer and Palliative Care Centre

Sarah Fisher, General Manager 01372 783400
Gill Avenue, Guildford, Surrey GU2 7WW

A specialist centre for patients and their families, affected by life-changing illnesses such as cancer, motor neurone disease, providing integrated, specialist, clinical and supportive complementary therapies to promote physical and emotional wellbeing

Therapies: Acupuncture, Aromatherapy, Art Therapy, Counselling, Indian Head (& Neck) Massage, Reflexology, Relaxation, Visualisation

Details: Available to clients, and to carers (except Acupuncture) on weekdays except Thursdays through professional referral. Different complementary therapies are available on a sessional basis at different times throughout the week – they are not all available during the times given. All therapies should be booked in advance. Patients and families are able to self-refer to the service, but undergo comprehensive assessment of need, and receive treatment against identified problems and agreed goals

Cost: All free of charge

Quality assurance: All complementary therapy practitioners are qualified healthcare professionals with a sound knowledge base of their subject and proven clinical skills. Clinical supervision is integral to good practice. Patients are fully assessed and problems identified prior to a therapy being offered. This ensures that treatment is given for an identified need against a planned and evaluated treatment goal

Materials supplied: A wide range of literature is available from our information centre, in addition to leaflets and professional resources

Promotion: Service leaflet; contact with the service; individual information leaflets about therapies offered

The Fountain Centre

Charlotte McDowell, Co-ordinator   **01483 406618**

St Luke's Cancer Centre, Royal Surrey County Hospital, Egerton Road, Guildford, Surrey GU2 7XX

The Fountain Centre is a charity working hand-in-hand with local hospital and social services

Therapies: Acupuncture, Aromatherapy, Art Therapy, Counselling, Herbal Remedies, Homeopathy, Massage, Nutritional Programmes, Reflexology, Reiki, Relaxation, Shiatsu, Therapeutic Touch

Details: All therapies are available to clients, and to carers (except Nutritional Programmes) on weekdays including Wednesday evenings through self referral. Aromatherapy, Art Therapy, Counselling, Massage, Reflexology, Reiki, Shiatsu and Therapeutic Touch are open to staff
All therapies should be advance booked but Reiki is available on a drop-in basis. Clients can be referred by health professionals for Counselling

Cost: Please enquire

Quality assurance: Understanding of patient's condition. Side effects of treatment. Complementary therapy consultation sheet

Materials supplied: The Centre has a library from which patients and their carers may borrow books, CDs, videos and cassettes

Promotion: Staff referrals; posters; leaflets; orientation evening; video

Surrey & Sussex Healthcare NHS Trust

Sue Quinn, Cancer/Palliative Care CNS   **01737 768511 x6685**
Cancer Nursing Services, East Surrey Hospital, Canada Avenue, Redhill, Surrey RH1 5RH

Therapies: Massage

Details: Available to clients, carers and staff on self referral (contact Surrey & Sussex Healthcare NHS Trust for availability). Advance booking is required

Cost: All free of charge

Quality assurance: Medical advice

Promotion: Word of mouth

Bournewood Community NHS Trust

Dr Bernadette Lee   **01932 826042**

Sam Beare Ward (Palliative Care Unit), Weybridge Hospital, Church Street, Weybridge, Surrey KT13 8DY

NHS specialist palliative care unit within a community hospital setting

Therapies:	Acupuncture, Aromatherapy, Counselling, Massage, Relaxation
Details:	All therapies are available to clients on Tuesdays, Thursdays and Fridays with Counselling also open to carers. Acupuncture requires professional referral but other therapies can be self referred. All therapies should be booked in advance
Cost:	All free of charge
Materials supplied:	Macmillan's Cancer Guide
Promotion:	Communication by direct referral

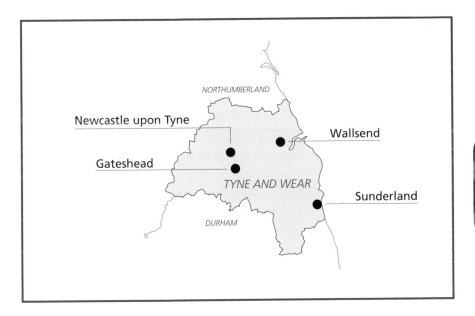

Complementary therapy services in
Tyne and Wear

Gateshead	● Gateshead Health NHS Trust
Newcastle	● Coping With Cancer North East
upon Tyne	● Marie Curie Cancer Care
	● Newcastle Primary Care Trust Specialist Palliative Care
	● St Oswald's Hospice
Sunderland	● Priority Healthcare Wearside NHS Trust
Wallsend	● Northumbria Healthcare NHS Trust

Gateshead Health NHS Trust

Ingrid Ablett-Spence, Lead Cancer Nurse   **0191 403 6095**
Queen Elizabeth Hospital, Trust Headquarters, Sheriff Hill, Gateshead, Tyne and Wear
NE9 6SX

Gateshead has a small inpatient palliative care unit that also provides day care

Therapies:	Acupuncture, Aromatherapy, Counselling, Massage, Reflexology, Relaxation
Details:	All therapies are available to clients with Counselling open to carers and staff, and Massage also open to staff (contact for details of availablity). Massage, Reflexology and Relaxation are available through self referral; Acupuncture requires professional referral
Cost:	Please enquire
Promotion:	Leaflets; useful information book

Coping With Cancer North East

Judith Woodroff, Manager of Volunteer Services   **01665 570068**
St. Joseph's Business Centre, West Lane, Killingworth, Newcastle upon Tyne, Tyne and
Wear NE12 0BH

The facility can be found across Tyne & Wear in chemotherapy day units, hospitals,
day hospices, breast surgery wards, GP surgeries and other settings

Therapies:	Aromatherapy, Art Therapy, Counselling, Massage, Reflexology, Reiki, Relaxation, Visualisation
Details:	All therapies are available to clients from Tuesday to Friday (including Wednesday evening) with Aromatherapy, Counselling, Massage, Reflexology, Reiki, Relaxation and Visualisation also open to carers, and Aromatherapy, Massage, Reflexology, Reiki, Relaxation and Visualisation open to staff, Drop-in for Art Therapy; book in advance for Aromatherapy, Counselling, Massage, Reflexology, Reiki, Relaxation,

Visualisation. Cancer patients are referred by healthcare professional but carers and staff can self-refer. A part-time complementary therapy co-ordinator is available

Cost: Please enquire

Quality assurance: Planning meeting with therapist covers treatments, side effects, etc. Complementary therapy guidelines in place to cover assessment procedures. All therapists MUST be members of relevant professional body and abide by their regulations

Materials supplied: Leaflets and consultation prior to booking for or taking up offer of therapy

Promotion: Leaflets; GP referrals; hospice literature; newsletters for volunteers and support groups

Marie Curie Cancer Care

Margaret Dobb, Caring Services Manager　　　　**0191 219 1000**
Marie Curie Centre, Marie Curie Drive, Newcastle upon Tyne, Tyne and Wear NE4 6SS

Provides inpatient, day care, outpatient and domiciliary services from a purpose-built unit

Therapies: Acupuncture, Aromatherapy, Counselling, Hypnotherapy/Hypnosis, Massage, Music Therapy, Reflexology, Relaxation, Visualisation

Details: All therapies are available to clients on all weekday afternoons and Monday/Friday mornings through professional referral. Therapies may be available over the weekend if trained nursing staff are on duty
Acupuncture, Aromatherapy, Counselling, Hypnotherapy/Hypnosis, Massage and Relaxation are open to carers and staff, with Reflexology additionally open to staff. Advance booking is required

Cost: All free of charge

Quality assurance: All therapists have to complete a questionnaire covering all aspects of their treatment. All therapists are interviewed and assessed in their given therapy. All patients are assessed daily as to the appropriateness of the therapy to be given

Promotion: Complementary therapies and general information leaflets; word of mouth; Posters around the centre

Newcastle Primary Care Trust Specialist Palliative Care Team

Lindsay Crack, Consultant   **0191 226 1315**
Arthurs Hill Clinic, Douglas Terrace, Newcastle upon Tyne, Tyne and Wear NE4 6BT

Therapies: Acupuncture, Hypnotherapy/Hypnosis, Massage, Reflexology

Details: All therapies are available to clients and carers through professional referral on Monday, Wednesday and Friday mornings with Acupuncture and Hypnotherapy/Hypnosis also open to staff

Cost: Please enquire

Quality assurance: Assessed by practitioner

Materials supplied: Cassettes for Hypnotherapy/Hypnosis and Relaxation.

Promotion: Word of mouth; contact and referral within the team; by district nurses attending teaching sessions

St Oswald's Hospice

Angela Egdell, Clinical Services Manager   **0191 285 0063**
Regent Avenue, Gosforth, Newcastle upon Tyne, Tyne and Wear NE1 3EE

St Oswald's provides inpatient, day hospice, day treatment and outpatient care

Therapies: Acupuncture, Aromatherapy, Massage, Reflexology, Relaxation

Details:	All therapies are available to clients and staff, with professional referral required for Acupuncture and self-referral for the remainder. All except Acupuncture are also available to carers. Open on Mondays, Tuesdays, Wednesday mornings, Thursdays, Friday mornings and Sunday mornings. Acupuncture can be booked in advance; drop-in available for the rest
Cost:	All free of charge
Quality assurance:	Following self-referral, patient discusses suitability of therapy with in-house medical team or GP. Training for all therapists in medical conditions, medication, etc. Full documentation of treatments given in patient's care plan
Promotion:	Included in information booklets; posters; annual reports

Priority Healthcare Wearside NHS Trust

Michael Walls, Project Co-ordinator **0191 516 6300**
Unit 30A, Business & Innovation Centre, Wearfields, Sunderland, Tyne and Wear
SR5 2TA

Offers complementary therapies to cancer patients and carers through a community-based project funded by the New Opportunites Fund for three years. This provision started on 1/11/01 as one element of 'Offering Options – Living with Cancer'

Therapies:	Aromatherapy, Counselling, Massage, Nutritional Programmes, Reflexology, Reiki, Shiatsu, Nutritional Supplements, Therapeutic Touch
Details:	Available to clients and carers on self referral, and can be referred by healthcare professional. Open on Mondays (including evenings), Tuesdays (including evenings) and Fridays (services available at other times and will develop further as demand increases). Advance booking is required
Cost:	All free of charge
Quality assurance:	Generally, referral is originated by healthcare professional, mainly GP, who has patient knowledge. At initial contact,

client is advised to discuss with GP/medical team. At extended initial session, client is interviewed to establish appropriateness

Materials supplied: 'Offering Options' leaflet, video available

Promotion: Leaflets; via existing relationships with health/social care professionals; advertising – local press/media coverage

Northumbria Healthcare NHS Trust

A P Waugh, Macmillan Clinical Nurse Specialist   **0191 220 5955**

Sir G B Hunter Memorial Hospital, The Green, Wallsend, Tyne and Wear NE28 7PB

The Trust's physical base is in the community, even if its organisational base is in the Trust's medical directorate

Therapies: Aromatherapy, Massage

Details: Available to clients on Tuesday and Thursday afternoons through professional referral

Cost: All free of charge

Quality assurance: Standards and protocols in place. Provided by Coping with Cancer registered practitioners

Promotion: Service not publicised; currently only available to day hospice patients

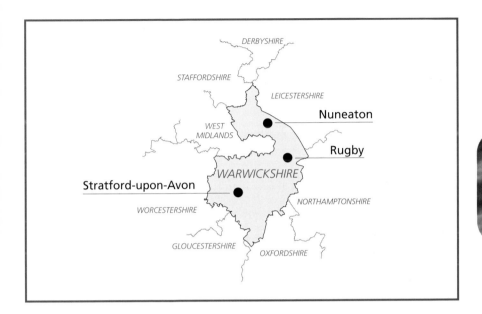

Complementary therapy services in

Warwickshire

Nuneaton	● Mary Ann Evans Hospice
Rugby	● British Association for Counselling
Stratford-upon-Avon	● The Shakespeare Hospice

Mary Ann Evans Hospice

Ann Hammond, Palliative Care Manager   **024 7686 5440**
George Eliot Hospital, College Street, Nuneaton, Warwickshire CV10 7QL

The hospice is based on an acute hospital site, which gives access to all departments. The facility has a partnership with North Warwickshire NHS Community Trust from which services are purchased

Therapies:	Aromatherapy, Art Therapy, Nutritional Supplements
Details:	Available to clients through professional referral except for Art Therapy (self referral). Contact for details of availability
Cost:	All free of charge
Quality assurance:	All patients assessed by aromatherapist prior to any treatment
Promotion:	Information given by hospice staff

British Association for Counselling

Information Service   **0807 443 5227**
1 Regent Place, Rugby, Warwickshire CV21 2PJ

The UK's major organisation for counselling, promoting, creating and maintaining good standards of practice, e.g. code of ethics, complaints procedure, accreditation schemes, etc. A list of local counsellors is available on request or from the website

Therapies:	Counselling
Details:	Available to clients, carers and staff on weekdays (08.45-17.00) through self referral
Cost:	A fee is charged for Counselling
Quality assurance:	The BAC offers a referral list via the Counselling and Psychotherapy Resources Directory. It also runs accreditation schemes for training and for individual counsellors
Promotion:	Internet – own website; leaflets

The Shakespeare Hospice

Kate Hall, Sister   **01789 266852**

Church Lane, Shottery, Stratford-upon-Avon, Warwickshire CV37 9UL

Therapies:	Aromatherapy, Art Therapy, Counselling, Massage, Meditation, Nutritional Programmes, Reflexology, Reiki, Relaxation, Nutritional Supplements
Details:	All therapies are available to clients from Monday to Thursday with Aromatherapy, Counselling, Massage, Meditation, Reflexology, Reiki and Relaxation open to carers, and Counselling available to staff. Professional referral is required for Aromatherapy, Art Therapy, Massage, Nutritional Programmes, Reflexology, Reiki and Nutritional Supplements; self referrals are accepted for Counselling, Meditation and Relaxation. Book in advance for Counselling, Nutritional Programmes and Nutritional Supplements; drop-in for other therapies
Cost:	All free of charge
Quality assurance:	Guidelines written on all treatments, including contra-indications. Consent forms completed. Always assessed by qualified nurse
Materials supplied:	Books, leaflets, audio cassettes and videos are available
Promotion:	Hospice leaflet; posters in GP surgeries; open day; newsletter

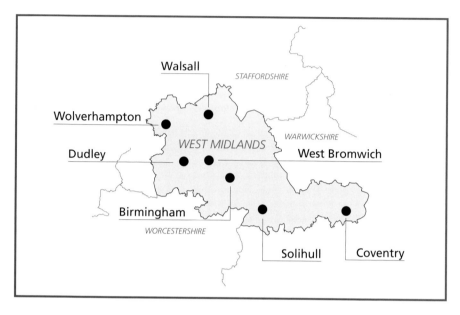

Complementary therapy services in
West Midlands

Birmingham	• Acorns Children's Hospice - Selly Oak
	• Birmingham Heartlands & Solihull NHS Hospitals Trust
	• Birmingham St Mary's Hospice
	• University Hospital Birmingham NHS Trust
Coventry	• Cancer Resource Centre
Dudley	• Cancer Support
Solihull	• Solihull Cancer Support Group
Walsall	• Little Bloxwich Day Hospice
	• Walsall Breast Cancer Self Help Group
	• Walsall Hospitals NHS Trust
West Bromwich	• Sandwell Healthcare NHS Trust
Wolverhampton	• Compton Hospice

Acorns Children's Hospice – Selly Oak

Mrs Anne Leung, Head Nurse   **0181 248 4850**
103 Oak Tree Lane, Selly Oak, Birmingham, West Midlands B29 6HZ

Offering care and support to children with life-limiting conditions up to the age of 19, and offering support to their families. Provides respite, emergency and terminal care in a home-from-home environment encompassing all needs

Therapies: Aromatherapy, Art Therapy, Counselling, Massage, Music Therapy, Reflexology, Nutritional Supplements
Details: All therapies are available to clients and carers all week on self referral, with Aromatherapy, Counselling, Massage and Reflexology open to staff
Cost: All free of charge
Quality assurance: Policy in place. Consent of family and/or child before therapy administered. Designated role for staff nurse who supervises other staff in use of oils
Materials supplied: Written information as requested – discussed with therapist
Promotion: When a child is accepted as a client, the community team worker explains the services

Birmingham Heartlands & Solihull NHS Hospitals Trust

Marjorie Small, Lead Cancer Nurse   **0121 424 2236**
Bordesley Green East, Bordesley Green, Birmingham, West Midlands B9 5SS

A haematology and oncology unit

Therapies: Reflexology, Relaxation, Nutritional Supplements
Details: All therapies are available to clients on Mondays to Fridays including evenings through self referral (professional referrals

for Nutritional Supplements also taken), with Reflexology and Relaxation open to carers. Book in advance for Reflexology and Relaxation; drop-in for Nutritional Supplements

Cost: All free of charge

Promotion: Leaflets; flyers; via support group

Birmingham St Mary's Hospice

Jan Jamieson, Complementary Therapy Co-ordinator　　　　**0121 472 1191**

176 Raddlebarn Road, Selly Park, Birmingham, West Midlands B29 7DA

Offers complementary therapy service to people with cancer (home care or outpatients), carers, bereaved relatives and staff

Therapies: Aromatherapy, Counselling, Massage, Reflexology, Reiki, Relaxation, Visualisation

Details: Available to clients, carers and staff Monday to Thursday and Friday afternoons through both professional and self referral (therapies may also be available *ad hoc* in the evenings). Book in advance for Aromatherapy, Massage, Reflexology, Reiki, Relaxation and Visualisation

Cost: All free of charge to clients and carers (charges apply for staff)

Quality assurance: Professionalism of therapists. If unsure, obtain resident doctor's permission

Materials supplied: Leaflets, after-care advice, relaxation tapes where appropriate

Promotion: Leaflet; word of mouth; referral

University Hospital Birmingham NHS Trust

Zoe Neary, Macmillan Clinical Nurse Specialist　　　**0121 472 1311　x3221**
Oak Tree Lane Offices, Selly Oak Hospital, Raddlebarn Road, Birmingham, West
Midlands B29 6JF

This entry is for our head and neck department, which provides care for patients with
a diagnosis of cancer

Therapies:	Aromatherapy, Counselling, Reflexology
Details:	Available to clients and carers on self referral (can be referred by healthcare professional). Counselling is available Monday to Wednesday. Reflexology and Aromatherapy are available on Friday mornings
Cost:	All free of charge
Quality assurance:	Discussed at multidisciplinary meetings. All team members giving complementary therapies are at clinical nurse specialist level in head and neck cancer nursing. Non-nurse therapists planned for the future will have clinical supervision from nurse specialist. Written information on side effects given to patients when gaining consent
Materials supplied:	Information leaflets, books, cassettes
Promotion:	Posters in all related departments – outpatients and wards; 'Get-a-head' website; 'Get-a-head' newsletter

Cancer Resource Centre

Alison Crichton, Information/Support Radiographer　　　**02476 538732**
Radiotherapy Department, Walsgrave General Hospital, Clifford Bridge Road,
Coventry, West Midlands CV2 2DX

The centre is based within the hospital's radiotherapy and oncology department

Therapies:	Aromatherapy, Counselling, Reflexology, Relaxation
Details:	All therapies are available to clients on self referral, with Relaxation open to carers and staff, and Counselling

additionally open to carers. Book in advance for Aromatherapy, Counselling and Reflexology; drop-in for Relaxation. Counselling is available Mondays, Wednesdays and Fridays. Reflexology is available on Monday afternoons and Friday mornings. Aromatherapy is available on Tuesdays. The centre is open from Monday to Friday (09.00-17.00)

Cost: All free of charge

Quality assurance: Patients informed by therapist about side effects, etc. and complete consent form and questionnaire. Therapists need to be registered with appropriate body and receive initial training from the Cancer Support Centre on the disease, treatments and side effects

Promotion: Posters and leaflets posted around the department; information booklets for patients receiving treatment

Cancer Support

Beverley Hart or Jaki Parrish   **01384 231232**
The White House, 10 Ednam Road, Dudley, West Midlands DY1 1JX

Provides practical help, emotional support and information for cancer patients and carers, and runs a drop-in information centre (open each weekday) and a 24-hour help line. Offers counselling/befriending, home/hospital visits, complementary therapies and group work

Therapies: Aromatherapy, Counselling, Massage, Indian Head (& Neck) Massage, Reflexology, Reiki

Details: Available to clients and carers on weekdays through self referral. Reflexology and Reiki are available at weekly branch group meetings in Brierley Hill and Halesowen. Book in advance for all therapies. (Patients and carers can be referred by healthcare professionals.)

Cost: All free of charge

Quality assurance: Consent form from GP or consultant required for any patient/carer receiving medical treatment. Therapists take full medical history at first appointment; list of contra-indications shown to client. Details of prescribed medication recorded; clients sign form confirming details they have provided

Materials supplied: Information centre has selection of books, printed material and videotapes on complementary therapies, and can offer guidance on reliable websites

Promotion: Information leaflets and posters; brochure; activities publicised in monthly newsletter and bi-annual contact magazine, 'Connect'; information displayed at local hospitals, libraries and community events

Solihull Cancer Support Group

Patricia or Shirley   **0121 711 1966 or 0121 705 1818**
c/o SIMTR, 1a Damson Parkway, Solihull, West Midlands B91 2PP

The support group is held in conference rooms

Therapies: Counselling, Meditation, Reflexology, Reiki, Relaxation, Spiritual Healing, Therapeutic Touch, Visualisation

Details: Available to clients and carers on Thursdays (19.30-22.30) through self referral

Cost: All free of charge

Quality assurance: All counsellors and healers are registered and hold insurance. All counsellors and healers will always give consultations and information

Materials supplied: Lending library, videos

Promotion: Leaflets; newsletters; advertising; word of mouth

Little Bloxwich Day Hospice

Elaine Cooper, Complementary Therapist   **01922 858735**

Stoney Lane, Little Bloxwich, Walsall, West Midlands WS3 3DW

The hospice's service is based at the day hospice; there is a clinic for outpatients and home visits are provided

Therapies:	Aromatherapy, Massage, Reflexology, Relaxation, Visualisation
Details:	Available to clients Monday to Friday mornings on self referral. Therapies available (each alternative week) on Tuesday and Wednesday afternoons. Advance booking is required
Cost:	All free of charge
Quality assurance:	Protocol/procedure – Massage, Aromatherapy, Reflexology. Referral criteria. GP informed
Promotion:	Leaflets; via Macmillan home care team/district nurses; via day hospice staff/medical directors

Walsall Breast Cancer Self Help Group

Jo Stackhouse, Chair and Group Co-ordinator   **01922 412731**

c/o 11 Wharwell Lane, Greater Wyrley, Walsall, West Midlands WS6 6ET

A voluntary organisation working alongside a breast surgeon/nurse on hospital clinic days, and part of the breast clinic team. The group has its own counselling room but also meets in the Trust's postgraduate centre and gives home visits if required

Therapies:	Counselling, Relaxation, Visualisation
Details:	Available to clients and carers on self referral. Counselling is available on Tuesday and Thursday mornings and Wednesday evenings (drop-in available)
Cost:	All free of charge
Promotion:	Via bi-monthly newsletter; word of mouth when we meet patients for the first time on breast clinic days

Walsall Hospitals NHS Trust

Josie Browne   **01922 721172 x 7168**
Trust Cancer Team, Moat Road, Walsall, West Midlands WS2 9PS

A chemotherapy unit within a district general hospital

Therapies:	Acupuncture, Aromatherapy, Massage, Reiki, Relaxation
Details:	Available to clients, carers and staff on Fridays through self referral. Book in advance for all therapies
Cost:	All free of charge
Quality assurance:	Therapist informed of patient's treatment, when last given and any side effects
Promotion:	Printed leaflets given to patients with cancer; verbal information given about complementary therapy service

Sandwell Healthcare NHS Trust

Lyn Spiers   **0121 607 7971**
2nd Floor Directorate Offices, Lyndon, West Bromwich, West Midlands B71 4HJ

The complementary therapy service operates from the newly opened Courtyard Centre, which is a Cancer Information & Support Service funded through Macmillan Cancer Relief

Therapies:	Aromatherapy, Massage, Reflexology
Details:	Available to clients on Mondays, Wednesdays and Fridays on self referral (can also be referred by a healthcare professional). Book in advance for all therapies
Cost:	All free of charge
Quality assurance:	Trust policy
Materials supplied:	Leaflets
Promotion:	Via clinical nurse specialists; posters; leaflets

Compton Hospice

Margaret Stone, Complementary Therapist   **01902 758151**

Compton Road West, Compton, Wolverhampton, West Midlands WV3 9DH

Offers inpatient and day care unit with community and hospital liaison teams

Therapies:	Aromatherapy, Massage, Reflexology
Details:	Available to clients and staff on weekdays except Wednesday through professional referral. Advance booking is required
Cost:	All free of charge
Quality assurance:	Patients are referred by health professional. Therapists discuss treatment options with patients and give feedback to referrer
Promotion:	Leaflets; home care/Macmillan service; recommendations from patients

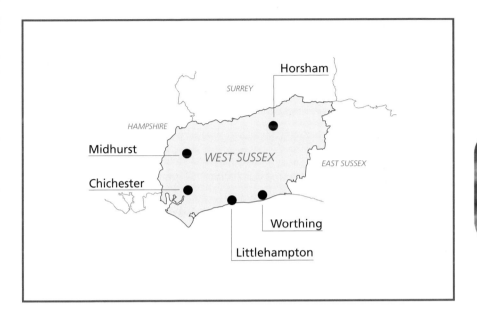

Complementary therapy services in

West Sussex

Chichester	• St. Wilfrid's Hospice
	• Wessex Cancer Help Centre
Horsham	• Crawley Cancer Contact
Littlehampton	• Cancer Support Group
Midhurst	• Midhurst Macmillan Specialist Palliative Care Service
Worthing	• Chestnut Tree House

St Wilfrid's Hospice

Alison Moorey   **01243 755802**
Grosvenor Road, Donnington, Chichester, West Sussex PO19 2FP

Runs three days a week; a 15-bedded inpatient unit with a day hospice and an
education centre, a comprehensive bereavement service and a community team
looking after 210 patients

Therapies:	Aromatherapy, Art Therapy, Counselling, Massage, Reflexology, Relaxation
Details:	All therapies are available to clients through professional referral with Aromatherapy, Art Therapy, Counselling, Massage and Reflexology open to carers, and Aromatherapy, Counselling, Massage and Reflexology open to staff. Runs on Tuesdays, Wednesdays and Fridays with Reflexology available on Thursday afternoons. (Complementary therapies are available at other times if a nurse with appropriate skills is free.) Book in advance. Note that the complementary therapy service offered to carers is on a limited basis
Cost:	All free of charge
Quality assurance:	Therapist makes a judgement based on information about the patient's condition
Promotion:	Leaflet for day hospice; information poster in inpatient unit; clinical nurse specialists inform patients; noticeboard and posters in day hospice

Wessex Cancer Help Centre

Mrs E A Deal, Co-ordinator   **01243 778516**
8 South Street, Chichester, West Sussex PO19 1EH

A resource centre with trained doctors and complementary therapists,
counsellors/befrienders and some ministers. The Centre works geographically which
allows it to cover a wider area, directing enquirers to a doctor, etc. nearest to them

Therapies:	Acupuncture, Aromatherapy, Chiropractic, Counselling, Herbal Remedies, Homeopathy, Massage, Meditation, Naturopathy, Osteopathy, Nutritional Programmes, Reflexology, Reiki, Relaxation, Shiatsu, Spiritual Healing, Nutritional Supplements, Therapeutic Touch, Visualisation
Details:	Available to clients, carers and staff through self referral. Drop-in for Counselling and Nutritional Supplements. Therapists have their own times and clinics
Cost:	Free of charge for Counselling There is a fee for Acupuncture, Aromatherapy, Chiropractic, Herbal Remedies, Homeopathy, Massage, Meditation, Naturopathy, Osteopathy, Nutritional Programmes, Reflexology, Reiki, Relaxation, Shiatsu, Spiritual Healing, Nutritional Supplements, Therapeutic Touch, Visualisation. All the practitioners are associated with the centre and charge their own fees
Quality assurance:	Individual therapists are responsible for this
Materials supplied:	Library, tapes and videos
Promotion:	Brochures; word of mouth; could be part of the discussion when we meet clients

Crawley Cancer Contact

Heather Goodare or Sue or Mike   **01403 261674/823858 or 01342 325538**
1 Heron Way, Horsham, West Sussex RH13 6DF

A self-help group offering support, information and complementary therapies for people with cancer and their families. Group meetings on Tuesday evenings (19.30–21.30) and 'drop-in' on Thursdays (14.00–18.00).

Therapies:	Acupuncture, Aromatherapy, Art Therapy, Counselling, Massage, Music Therapy, Reflexology, Reiki, Relaxation, Spiritual Healing, Therapeutic Touch, Visualisation

Details:	Available to clients, carers and staff on Tuesday evenings and Thursday afternoons through self referral. Counselling is arranged at mutually convenient times. Occasionally there are Saturday morning workshops. Book in advance for Acupuncture, Aromatherapy, Art Therapy, Counselling, Massage, Music Therapy, Reflexology, Reiki and Spiritual Healing; drop-in for Reiki, Relaxation, Therapeutic Touch and Visualisation. Nutritional information is also available
Cost:	All free of charge. After eight sessions of Counselling or ten sessions of other therapies a donation is requested to cover costs
Quality assurance:	We have regular team meetings of complementary therapists to discuss these issues. All therapists are offered appropriate support
Materials supplied:	Group library has many volumes on complementary therapies. Relaxation tapes available
Promotion:	Leaflet and poster, presentation at local hospitals

Cancer Support Group

Ivy Nicholson or Rosemary Isherwood   **01903 719804 or 01243 585446**

Littlehampton Natural Health Centre, 10c Granville Road, Littlehampton, West Sussex BN17 5JU

Complementary therapies are provided at the centre

Therapies:	Acupuncture, Aromatherapy, Chiropractic, Herbal Remedies, Homeopathy, Massage, Music Therapy, Osteopathy, Reflexology, Reiki, Shiatsu, Spiritual Healing, Nutritional Supplements
Details:	Available to clients and carers through self referral, Monday to Saturday, including Monday evenings (also sometimes available on other evenings). Drop-in for Reiki and Spiritual Healing therapies. Clients can be referred by health professionals
Cost:	Free of charge for Reflexology, Reiki, Spiritual Healing

There is a fee for Acupuncture, Aromatherapy, Chiropractic, Herbal Remedies, Homeopathy, Massage, Music Therapy, Osteopathy, Shiatsu, Nutritional Supplements

Quality assurance: Left to individual therapists
Materials supplied: Books and tapes on cancer care
Promotion: Leaflets and posters

Midhurst Macmillan Specialist Palliative Care Service

Sue Bowen, Clinical Services Manager   **01730 811121**
King Edward VII Hospital, Midhurst, West Sussex GU29 0BL

Complementary therapies are provided by volunteer complementary therapists for inpatients only if they have been referred through a professional

Therapies: Aromatherapy, Massage
Details: Available to clients on Monday, Wednesday and Friday afternoons on professional referral
Cost: All free of charge
Quality assurance: Patient information and consent form. Documentation from referring professional to volunteer therapist is held in patient's notes
Promotion: This service is ward-based only. It is referred to in the inpatient directory of services and guidelines for patients

Chestnut Tree House

Kate Barker, Director of Children's Services   **01903 837031**

Columbia House, Columbia Drive, Worthing, West Sussex BN13 3DD

A paediatric palliative care service for young people up to the age of 24 which includes respite/symptom management and terminal care. A community-based hospice opens in Spring 2003

Therapies:	Aromatherapy, Art Therapy, Massage, Meditation, Music Therapy, Reflexology, Relaxation, Spiritual Healing, Visualisation
Details:	All therapies are available to clients and staff through self referral, with Aromatherapy, Massage, Meditation, Reflexology, Relaxation and Visualisation open to carers. Open on Mondays, Tuesday mornings, Wednesdays (including evenings), Fridays (including evenings). Book in advance for all therapies
Cost:	All free of charge
Quality assurance:	Health and safety legislation. Consultation and discussion. Consent. Evaluation
Promotion:	Leaflets; posters; web news; information sheets; open days

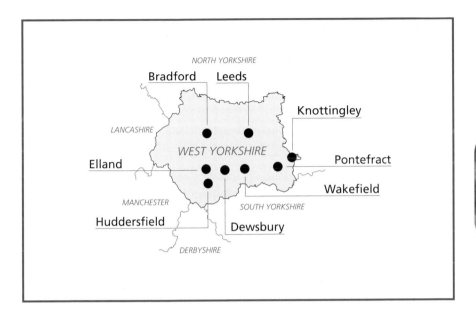

Complementary therapy services in

West Yorkshire

Bradford	● Bradford Cancer Support
	● Bradford Hospitals NHS Trust
	● Marie Curie Cancer Care
Dewsbury	● Rosewood Centre
Elland	● Overgate Hospice
Huddersfield	● Kirkwood Hospice
Knottingley	● Castleford & District C.S.H.G.
Leeds	● Robert Ogden Macmillan Centre
	● St Gemma's Hospice
Pontefract	● Pontefract and Pinderfields NHS Trust
	● The Prince of Wales Hospice
Wakefield	● Pinderfields General Hospital

Bradford Cancer Support

Alison Blundell   **01274 776688**

Daisy Bank, 109 Duckworth Lane, Bradford, West Yorkshire BD9 6RN

The facility runs a range of services to help patients and carers cope with cancer at all stages of the disease. As well as complementary therapies, transport, welfare benefits advice and various groups (support, Asian women, luncheon) are offered free of charge

Therapies:	Aromatherapy, Art Therapy, Counselling, Massage, Reflexology, Reiki, Relaxation, Visualisation
Details:	All therapies are available to clients and carers through self referral on Mondays, Tuesdays, Wednesday afternoons, Thursday afternoons and Friday mornings. Aromatherapy, Art Therapy, Counselling, Massage, Reflexology and Reiki are open to staff. Advance booking is required
Cost:	All free of charge There is a charge for Art Therapy for staff
Quality assurance:	On referral, each client's hospital consultant and GP will be notified and consent obtained. All therapists supervised by complementary therapies co-ordinator, a trained nurse working at centre and in a hospice
Materials supplied:	Centre leaflet and books; videos available on loan
Promotion:	Centre booklet and leaflets; cancer directories; information centre based in Bradford Royal Infirmary; hospital staff, GPs and specialist nurses will also make clients aware of complementary therapies

Bradford Hospitals NHS Trust

Pat Mowatt, Macmillan Nurse, Palliative Care Team   **01274 364035**

Bradford Royal Infirmary, Duckworth Lane, Bradford, West Yorkshire BD9 6RJ

An acute hospital site split over two sites: Bradford Royal Infirmary and St Luke's Hospital

Therapies:	Aromatherapy, Massage, Reflexology
Details:	Available to clients on Wednesday afternoons through self referral
Cost:	All free of charge
Quality assurance:	Essential oils are not used for Massage if chemotherapy is in progress
Materials supplied:	Cancer Support Centre's booklet about their complementary therapy services
Promotion:	Promoted verbally to inpatients on oncology and haematology wards where complementary therapies are used. Complementary therapy service for patients and carers offered by, and mentioned in booklets from, Cancer Support Centre which is a voluntary organisation located near the Bradford Royal Infirmary (BRI). Booklets available throughout Trust and at our soon-to-be-open Cancer Information Centre at the BRI

Marie Curie Cancer Care

Christine Matthews, Day Therapy Leader   **01274 337000**
Marie Curie Centre – Bradford, Maudsley Street, Bradford, West Yorkshire BD3 9LH

Therapies:	Acupuncture, Aromatherapy, Art Therapy, Counselling, Massage, Reflexology, Reiki, Therapeutic Touch
Details:	All therapies are available to clients on Mondays, Wednesdays and Thursdays through professional referral, with Counselling, Reiki and Therapeutic Touch available to carers, and with Acupuncture, Aromatherapy, Counselling, Reflexology, Reiki and Therapeutic Touch open to staff. Book in advance for all therapies
Cost:	All free of charge
Quality assurance:	Assessment and monitoring by medical and nursing staff
Materials supplied:	Leaflets on each therapy given prior to treatment
Promotion:	Patient information leaflets. Word of mouth via palliative care teams in hospitals and community trusts

Rosewood Centre

Sarah Wright   **01924 512039**
Palliative Day Care Centre, Dewsbury & District Hospital, Halifax Road, Dewsbury,
West Yorkshire WF13 4HS

The centre offers physical, social and psychological support to patients with palliative
care needs

Therapies:	Aromatherapy, Art Therapy
Details:	Available to clients on Tuesdays and Wednesdays through professional referral. Advance booking is required
Cost:	All free of charge
Quality assurance:	Assessment by aromatherapist prior to offering therapy. Protocols in place
Promotion:	Promoting service by word of mouth (new service in developmental stage). Service introduced on a one-to-one basis, describing therapies and their uses

Overgate Hospice

Jenni Feather, Matron   **01422 379151**
30 Hullen Edge Road, Elland, West Yorkshire HX5 0QY

An independent hospice with 12 beds also providing day hospice care four days a
week and serving a population of 190,000

Therapies:	Aromatherapy, Art Therapy, Counselling, Massage, Meditation, Relaxation, Therapeutic Touch
Details:	All therapies are available through professional referral to clients on Mondays, Tuesday afternoons, Thursdays, and Friday afternoons, with Aromatherapy, Counselling, Massage and Therapeutic Touch open to carers and Counselling and Meditation open to staff
Cost:	All free of charge
Quality assurance:	Professional assessment; protocols; leaflets
Promotion:	Leaflets; on arrival at hospice/day hospice

Kirkwood Hospice

John D Murgatroyd, Matron   **01484 557900**
21 Albany Road, Dalton, Huddersfield, West Yorkshire HD5 9UY

Kirkwood comprises an inpatient unit, a day care centre, two outreach day care centres, bereavement services (including children) which are available to the wider community, and an education centre linked to the local university

Therapies:	Aromatherapy, Art Therapy, Counselling, Massage, Meditation, Reflexology, Reiki, Relaxation, Spiritual Healing, Visualisation
Details:	Available to clients, carers and staff on weekdays (therapies are available at weekends by special arrangement) through self referral. Advance booking is required; clients can also be referred by healthcare professionals (drop-in services are also being considered)
Cost:	All free of charge
Quality assurance:	Full assessment prior to commencement of therapy
Materials supplied:	Taped cassettes and literature
Promotion:	Patient/health professional information leaflets; talks to lay and professional groups; educational sessions and workshops

Castleford & District C.S.H.G

Fred Walker, Secretary   **01977 675644**
47 Windermere Drive, Knottingley, West Yorkshire WF11 0ND

A community-based organisation meeting formally on the third Wednesday of each month in a community setting

Therapies:	Aromatherapy, Art Therapy, Drama Therapy, Massage, Reflexology, Reiki, Relaxation, Spiritual Healing, Visualisation
Details:	All therapies are available to clients on weekdays through self referral, with Aromatherapy, Art Therapy, Massage, Reflexology, Reiki, Relaxation, Spiritual Healing and Visualisation also open to carers. Advance booking is required

Cost:	All free of charge
Quality assurance:	A professional takes down details before appointments to ensure the safety of patients and carers. Clients then receive booklets
Materials supplied:	Relaxation tapes; library with comprehensive information in multimedia format
Promotion:	Leaflets; speakers; newsletters; personal recommendations; word of mouth from other patients

Robert Ogden Macmillan Centre

Dorothy Lambeth or Jane Henderson   **0113 2066498**

St. James's University Hospital, Beckett Street, Leeds, West Yorkshire LS9 7TF

Operated from a purpose-built cancer information and support centre

Therapies:	Aromatherapy, Art Therapy, Reflexology, Reiki, Spiritual Healing, Therapeutic Touch
Details:	All therapies are available to clients on weekdays, with Art Therapy, Reflexology, Reiki, Spiritual Healing and Therapeutic Touch also open to carers. Self referrals are accepted for all complementary therapies except Aromatherapy. Advance booking is required
Cost:	All free of charge
Quality assurance:	Full information available to staff and patients
Materials supplied:	Books and videos are available from the Centre library; everyone is given an appropriate leaflet
Promotion:	Leaflets and posters

St Gemma's Hospice

Marianne Tavares, Complementary Therapies Co-ordinator   **0113 218 5500**
Harrogate Road, Moortown, Leeds, West Yorkshire LS17 6QD

Specialist palliative care

Therapies:	Aromatherapy, Counselling, Massage, Meditation, Reiki, Relaxation, Visualisation
Details:	Aromatherapy, Counselling, Massage, Reiki, Relaxation and Visualisation are available to clients and carers on Mondays, Tuesdays, Wednesday and Friday afternoons, with Aromatherapy, Massage, Meditation and Reiki also open to staff. Self referral accepted for Aromatherapy, Counselling, Massage, Reiki, Relaxation and Visualisation. Clients can be referred by healthcare professionals. Creative arts therapy is also provided
Cost:	All free of charge
Quality assurance:	The patient is discussed within the clinical team and assessed by the complementary therapies co-ordinator or designated therapists. For Counselling, social workers provide the service and conduct the assessment
Promotion:	Hospice information booklet; multidisciplinary clinical team

Pontefract and Pinderfields NHS Trust

Mrs B J Greatorex   **01977 606170**
Friarwood Lane, Pontefract General Infirmary, Pontefract, West Yorkshire WF8 1PL

Therapies:	Acupuncture, Aromatherapy, Counselling, Massage, Nutritional Programmes, Relaxation, Nutritional Supplements
Details:	All therapies are available to clients on Mondays, Tuesday mornings, Wednesdays and Fridays (at times to suit clients), with Counselling also available to carers. Self referrals are accepted for Counselling; professional referral required for Acupuncture, Nutritional Programmes, Relaxation and

Nutritional Supplements. Advance booking required for Aromatherapy, Massage and Relaxation. Complementary therapy is available via advance booking for carers of cancer patients at the two hospices within the catchment area

Cost: All free of charge

Quality assurance: Part of care pathway. Verbal information on side effects

Materials supplied: Provided through the hospices for patients and carers. No specific literature available within the cancer unit

Promotion: Holistic referrals

The Prince of Wales Hospice

Julie Cade, Patient Services Director   **01977 708868**

Halfpenny Lane, Pontefract, West Yorkshire WF8 4BG

Therapies: Acupuncture, Aromatherapy, Art Therapy, Counselling, Drama Therapy, Massage, Meditation, Music Therapy, Reflexology, Reiki, Relaxation, Shiatsu, Spiritual Healing, Visualisation

Details: Available to clients, carers and staff on professional referral (Acupuncture, Counselling) and self referral (Aromatherapy, Art Therapy, Drama Therapy, Massage, Meditation, Music Therapy, Reflexology, Reiki, Relaxation, Shiatsu, Spiritual Healing, Visualisation). Aromatherapy, Massage and Relaxation are available on Mondays (for carers only) and Wednesdays. Reiki is available on Tuesdays and Fridays (patients and staff only) plus Wednesdays. Spiritual Healing therapy is available on Wednesdays

Cost: Please enquire

Quality assurance: Assessment; information; record-keeping; clinical supervision

Materials supplied: Booklet and video

Promotion: Posters; leaflets; booklets; included in local directory of palliative care services; video

Pinderfields General Hospital

Lynette Humphries   **01924 212290**
Aberford Road, Wakefield, West Yorkshire WF1 4DG

Within the department of palliative medicine, Pinderfields covers both Pontefract General Infirmary and Pinderfields (Wakefield) General Hospital. It only covers the community in the Wakefield side of the district

Therapies:	Counselling, Relaxation
Details:	Provides Counselling for clients, and Counselling and Relaxation for carers on Wednesdays and Thursdays through self referral. Advance booking required
Cost:	All free of charge
Materials supplied:	Relaxation tapes
Promotion:	Leaflets explaining the bereavement support service for relatives and carers

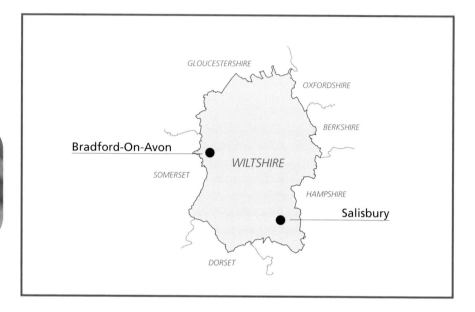

Complementary therapy services in

Wiltshire

| **Bradford-On-Avon** | • Dorothy House Hospice Care |
| **Salisbury** | • Salisbury District Hospital |

Dorothy House Hospice Care

Lynne Churchman, Director of Nursing　　　　　　**01225 722988**
Winsley, Bradford-On-Avon, Wiltshire BA15 2LE

Therapies:	Aromatherapy, Massage, Reflexology, Relaxation
Details:	Therapies available on Monday afternoons (at other times on an individual basis), either at the hospice or in the community. All therapies are available through professional referral to clients with Relaxation also open to carers
Cost:	All free of charge
Quality assurance:	Clinical co-ordinator co-ordinates therapists and patients seen
Promotion:	Leaflet; day care; nurse specialists; assessment unit; all professionals involved in our service

Salisbury District Hospital

Miss Jane Bailey, Junior Sister　　　　　　**01722 336262 x2113**
Oldstock Road, Salisbury, Wiltshire SP2 8BJ

Therapies:	Aromatherapy, Art Therapy, Counselling, Drama Therapy, Massage, Music Therapy, Reflexology
Details:	All therapies are available to clients on professional referral, with Aromatherapy, Counselling and Massage also open to carers, and Reflexology open to carers and staff. Reflexology is available on weekdays (9.00–16.00); contact for availability of other therapies
Cost:	All free of charge
Quality assurance:	Contra-indications for each therapy. Policy. Doctor's signature. Therapy assessment
Promotion:	Through day support unit; leaflets and booklet; on admission to the hospice

257

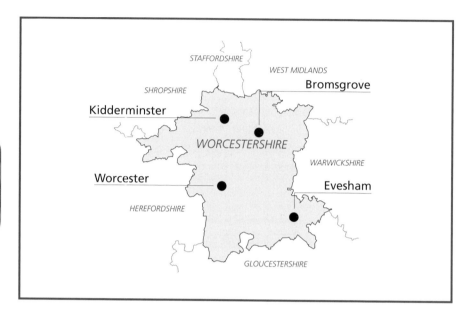

Complementary therapy services in

Worcestershire

Bromsgrove	• Primrose Hospice & Cancer Help Centre
Evesham	• Evesham Community Hospital
Kidderminster	• Kemp Hospice
	• Worcestershire Acute Hospitals NHS Trust
Worcester	• St Richard's Hospice
	• Worcestershire Acute Hospitals NHS Trust

Primrose Hospice & Cancer Help Centre

Veronica Bratt, Complementary Therapy Co-ordinator   **01527 871051**

St Godwald's Road, Finstall, Bromsgrove, Worcestershire B60 3BW

An independent charity working alongside other agencies, offering an advisory and support service to mainly cancer patients, their families and friends

Therapies:	Aromatherapy, Art Therapy, Bowen Technique, Homeopathy, Massage, Indian Head (& Neck) Massage, Reflexology, Reiki, Relaxation, Therapeutic Touch, Visualisation
Details:	All therapies are available on self referral to clients and to carers (except Art Therapy and Homeopathy). Operates on Monday mornings, Tuesdays, Wednesdays, Thursday and Friday mornings. Advance book for Aromatherapy, Bowen Technique, Homeopathy, Massage, Indian Head (& Neck) Massage, Reflexology, Reiki and Therapeutic Touch; drop-in for Art Therapy, Relaxation and Visualisation
Cost:	All free of charge
Quality assurance:	Full but very gentle treatments are offered to all patients. Indian Head (& Neck) Massage is not offered to patients who are in a frail condition. A complementary therapy policy is in place with clinical guidelines. Patient assessment form
Materials supplied:	Leaflets
Promotion:	Leaflets; verbal communication to healthcare professionals in hospital and community services; presentations to lay people; local media and fundraising activities

Evesham Community Hospital

Karen Chilver, Macmillan Nurse   **01386 502403**

Macmillan Unit, Waterside, Evesham, Worcestershire WR11 6JT

Provides specialist palliative care with hospice beds in a community hospital

Therapies:	Acupuncture, Aromatherapy, Counselling, Massage, Nutritional Programmes, Reflexology, Nutritional Supplements
Details:	All therapies are available to clients on either professional or self referral, with Counselling also open to carers and staff. Appointments are booked to suit patients and those offering the service
Cost:	All free of charge
Quality assurance:	Clients can self-refer, but treatment would have to be approved by doctor or healthcare professional
Promotion:	Leaflet; information given on admission

Kemp Hospice

Helen Windridge, Nurse Manager   **01562 861217**

58 Sutton Park Road, Kidderminster, Worcestershire DY11 6LF

A day hospice

Therapies:	Aromatherapy, Counselling, Massage, Reflexology, Relaxation, Nutritional Supplements
Details:	All therapies are available to clients on weekdays (afternoons by appointment) on professional referral. Aromatherapy, Counselling, Massage and Reflexology are also open to carers and Aromatherapy, Massage and Reflexology are open to staff. Advance booking is required for Aromatherapy, Massage, Reflexology and Relaxation
Cost:	Please enquire
Quality assurance:	Discussion about therapy and consent signed
Materials supplied:	Relaxation tapes
Promotion:	Information leaflet; talk to patients about services available

Worcestershire Acute Hospitals NHS Trust

Trish Wheal, Macmillan Clinical Nurse Specialist   **01562 823424 x3802**

Kidderminster General Hospital, Millbrook Suite, Bewdley Road, Kidderminster,
Worcestershire DY11 6RJ

Provides complementary therapies within the Millbrook Suite for both oncology and
palliative patients

Therapies:	Aromatherapy, Reflexology, Relaxation
Details:	Available to clients and carers Monday to Wednesday and on Thursday mornings, through self referral. Advance booking is required
Cost:	All free of charge
Promotion:	Posters; leaflets; direct contact via clinics

St Richard's Hospice

Rachel Bucknall, Care Director   **01905 763963**

Rose Hill, Worcester, Worcestershire WR5 1EY

St Richard's offers a day hospice, a home care team and an education and resource
centre

Therapies:	Aromatherapy, Art Therapy, Homeopathy, Massage, Music Therapy, Reflexology, Reiki, Relaxation, Nutritional Supplements, Therapeutic Touch, Visualisation
Details:	All therapies are available to clients on weekdays through professional referral. Additionally, Aromatherapy, Massage, Reflexology and Visualisation are available to carers
Cost:	Free of charge for Aromatherapy, Art Therapy, Massage, Music Therapy, Reflexology, Relaxation, Nutritional Supplements, Therapeutic Touch, Visualisation There is a fee for Homeopathy, Reiki
Quality assurance:	Policy and procedure in place
Promotion:	Discussed with patients/families after being referred to the service. Leaflets

Worcestershire Acute Hospitals NHS Trust

Pat Wainwright   **01905 760158**
Chemotherapy Unit, Castle Street Branch, Castle Street, Worcester WR1 3AS

Only open to patients receiving chemotherapy at Worcester (due to workload and funding restrictions)

Therapies:	Aromatherapy, Massage
Details:	Therapies are available to clients, carers and staff on Tuesday and Thursday mornings through professional or self referral
Cost:	All free of charge
Quality assurance:	On discussion with a healthcare professional
Materials supplied:	Information leaflets
Promotion:	Leaflets; verbally at pre-chemotherapy clinics

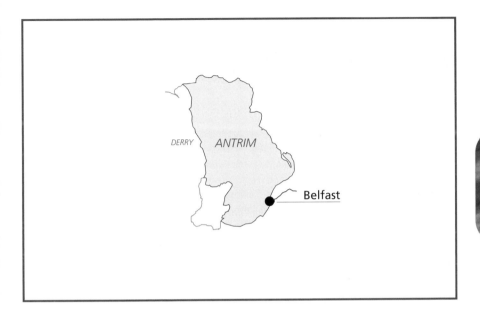

Complementary therapy services in

Antrim

Belfast
- Action Cancer
- Marie Curie Cancer Care Belfast
- The Gerard Lynch Centre
- Ulster Hospital

Action Cancer

Mary Connolly/Marita McMullan   **02890 244200**
1 Marlborough Park, Belfast, Antrim BT9 6XS

As a charity, Action Cancer provides, among other things, information/support services for cancer patients and their families. It also offers complementary therapies not only on its own premises, but on the oncology and haematology wards of Belfast City Hospital

Therapies:	Aromatherapy, Counselling, Massage, Meditation, Reflexology, Reiki, Relaxation, Therapeutic Touch, Visualisation, Yoga
Details:	Available to clients, carers and staff on weekdays through self referral. Book in advance for Aromatherapy, Counselling, Massage, Meditation, Reflexology, Reiki, Relaxation, Therapeutic Touch and Visualisation; drop-in for Yoga. Support groups for both men and women are available
Cost:	All free of charge
Quality assurance:	Require doctor's signature for cancer patients who request complementary therapy. Therapists specially trained to adapt treatment to each client. Therapists specially trained in cancer care when using Aromatherapy, Reflexology and Therapeutic Touch
Materials supplied:	Relaxation cassettes
Promotion:	Leaflets; posters; advertising; offering complementary therapy services on oncology and haematology wards of Belfast City Hospital

Marie Curie Cancer Care – Belfast

Alison Pollock, Senior Physiotherapist   **028 9079 4200**
Kensington Road, Belfast, Antrim BT5 6NF

A 19-bedded specialist palliative care unit

Therapies:	Acupuncture, Aromatherapy, Art Therapy, Counselling,

Massage, Music Therapy, Reflexology, Relaxation, Therapeutic Touch, Visualisation

Details: All therapies are available to clients on Monday afternoons, Wednesdays, and Friday mornings through professional referral. Aromatherapy, Massage, Reflexology and Therapeutic Touch are also open to carers and staff with Counselling and Relaxation additionally open to carers

Cost: Please enquire

Quality assurance: Referrals are channelled through a complementary therapy qualified health professional who then passes the information on to the volunteer therapists

Promotion: Word of mouth

The Gerard Lynch Centre

Lyn Lamont, Head of Complementary Therapy　　　　**028 9069 8202**
Belvoir Park Hospital, Belfast, Antrim BT8 8JR

A drop-in centre in the grounds of Belvoir Park Hospital with contemporary non-hospital décor. Facilities include: easy car parking, meeting room, internet access, library. Specialist facilities for complementary therapies

Therapies: Aromatherapy, Art Therapy, Counselling, Homeopathy, Hypnotherapy/Hypnosis, Massage, Meditation, Reflexology, Relaxation, T'ai Chi, Therapeutic Touch, Visualisation

Details: All therapies are available to clients on weekdays and Tuesday evenings, with Counselling, Hypnotherapy/Hypnosis, Meditation, Relaxation, T'ai Chi and Visualisation also open to carers, and Counselling, Meditation and T'ai Chi available to staff. All therapies may be self referred but Aromatherapy, Counselling, Massage, Reflexology and Therapeutic Touch are also open to professional referrals. Drop-in for Hypnotherapy/Hypnosis, Meditation, Relaxation, T'ai Chi and Visualisation; advance booking required for Aromatherapy, Art

265

Therapy, Counselling, Homeopathy, Massage, Reflexology and Therapeutic Touch.

Cost: Please enquire

Quality assurance: Guidelines for staff on patient referral for clinical psychology, Counselling and complementary therapies. Guide letters to GPs

Materials supplied: CancerBACUP, Bristol Cancer Help Centre video and information. Selection of books, internet access

Promotion: Leaflets and posters; letters to consultants/GPs; City Hospital Trust website; newspaper, TV and radio features; networking with our voluntary/charity organisations

Ulster Hospital

Alison Porter, Macmillan Senior Nurse　　　　　　　　**028 9056 4810**

Upper Newtownards Road, Dundonald, Belfast, Antrim BT161RH

The hospital's cancer unit provides site-specific cancer care with an on-site chemotherapy unit

Therapies: Aromatherapy, Counselling, Massage, Relaxation, Nutritional Supplements, Therapeutic Touch

Details: All therapies are available to clients, with Counselling also open to carers, through professional referral (Nutritional Supplements) and self referral (Aromatherapy, Counselling, Massage, Relaxation, Therapeutic Touch). Open on Tuesday afternoons; book in advance for all therapies; drop-in for Counselling

Cost: All free of charge

Quality assurance: Patients self-refer, but permission is sought from relevant consultant or GP. Through qualifications obtained and draft hospital policy in progress

Materials supplied: Information leaflet on Aromatherapy

Promotion: Personal communication – provided only within the chemotherapy unit

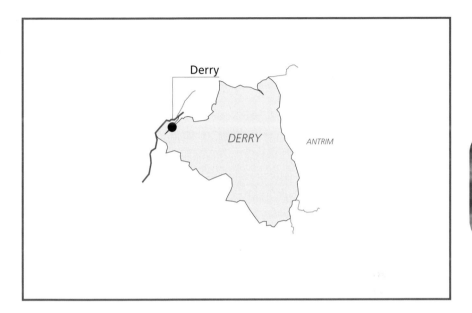

Complementary therapy services in

Derry

Derry   ● Derry Well Woman Centre

Derry Well Woman Centre

Bridie Gallagher   028 71360777
17 Queen Street, Derry BT48 7EQ

A voluntary women's health organisation

Therapies:	Aromatherapy, Counselling, Herbal Remedies, Homeopathy, Massage, Meditation, Nutritional Programmes, Reflexology, Reiki, Relaxation, Spiritual Healing, Nutritional Supplements, Therapeutic Touch, Visualisation
Details:	All therapies are available to clients on self referral with Counselling also open to carers. Runs on Tuesdays, Wednesday evenings, Thursday afternoons and Friday mornings. There are also support groups every fortnight (on Friday mornings) and a two-day cancer programme in January and April/May. Advance booking is required
Cost:	All free of charge. Therapies offered as part of 'Well Woman' programme
Quality assurance:	All practitioners fully trained and have nursing background. Based on information provided, all clients can assess appropriateness of each service. Maintain links with Belvoir Park and AHSST Cancer Unit to ensure complementary therapies complement traditional treatments. All programmes supported by access to cancer support group – facilitated by health visitor and nurse
Materials supplied:	Handouts on essential oils – use and contra-indications and meditation, relaxation tapes
Promotion:	Information leaflets; programme booklets; public notices; newspaper advertising; local radio

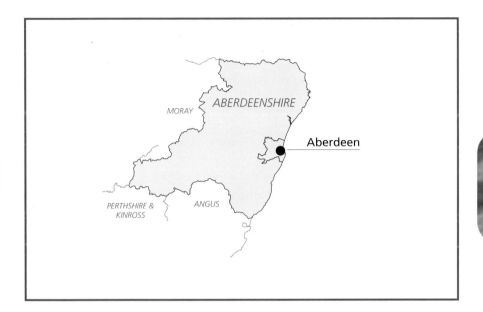

Complementary therapy services in
Aberdeenshire

Aberdeen   • CLAN (Cancer Link Aberdeen & North)

CLAN (Cancer Link Aberdeen & North)

Debbie Thomson, Centre Manager   **01224 647000**

Cancer Support Centre, CLAN House, Caroline Place, Aberdeen, Aberdeenshire AB25 2TH

An Aberdeen-based charity open to anyone, their carers or families in Grampian, Orkney or Shetland who is affected by cancer. The centre offers support, information and a range of complementary therapies

Therapies:	Aromatherapy, Art Therapy, Counselling, Reflexology, Reiki, Relaxation, Spiritual Healing, Visualisation
Details:	All therapies are available to clients and carers on weekdays through self referral. Relaxation and Visualisation are also open to staff. Book in advance for Aromatherapy, Reflexology, Reiki and Spiritual Healing therapies; drop-in for Art Therapy, Counselling, Relaxation and Visualisation
Cost:	All free of charge
Quality assurance:	All therapists fully qualified and experienced, the majority with nursing/paramedical backgrounds. Information leaflets available on all therapies
Materials supplied:	Information leaflets, books on complementary therapies in our library, relaxation/visualisation tapes, videos
Promotion:	Posters at hospitals, clinics, Macmillan nurses; press/media; website; 'Guide to CLAN Cancer Support centre' booklet; leaflets on individual therapies

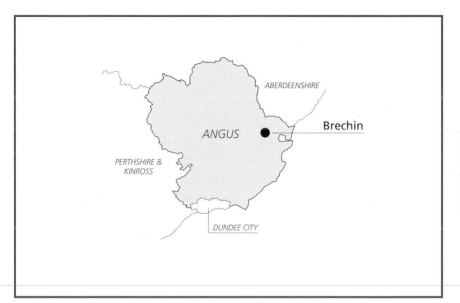

Complementary therapy services in

Angus

Brechin   ● Stracathro Hospital Macmillan Centre

Stracathro Hospital Macmillan Centre

Anne Pender   **01356 665014**
Brechin, Angus DD9 7QA

A palliative day care centre in grounds of Stracathro Hospital

Therapies:	Acupuncture, Aromatherapy, Art Therapy, Hypnotherapy/Hypnosis, Massage, Reflexology, Reiki, Relaxation, Therapeutic Touch
Details:	All therapies are available to clients on weekdays through self referral (or professional referral for Hypnotherapy/Hypnosis). Reiki is available on Tuesdays and Wednesdays; Reflexology on Thursdays and Therapeutic Touch on Fridays. Advance booking is required
Cost:	Please enquire
Quality assurance:	Consent is obtained from medical practitioner/person with clinical responsibility. Full assessment is carried out and documented and a treatment plan and outcomes are documented
Materials supplied:	Extensive book, audio and video cassette library
Promotion:	Written information; when patients are assessed for specialist palliative day care – complementary therapies are described

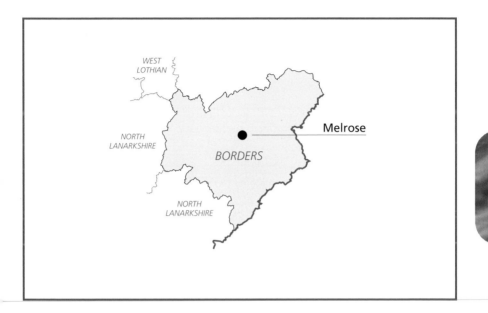

Complementary therapy services in

Borders

Melrose   • Borders General Hospital NHS Trust

Borders General Hospital NHS Trust

Elaine Peace, Macmillan Lead Cancer Nurse   **01896 826825**
Borders General Hospital, Melrose, Borders TD6 9BS

Therapies:	Relaxation, Nutritional Supplements
Details:	Available to clients on Mondays, Wednesday mornings and Fridays through professional referral
Cost:	All free of charge
Quality assurance:	Assessment made by professional involved. Nutrition/dietician is part of palliative care team and will assess nutritional state and supplement use
Promotion:	Word of mouth

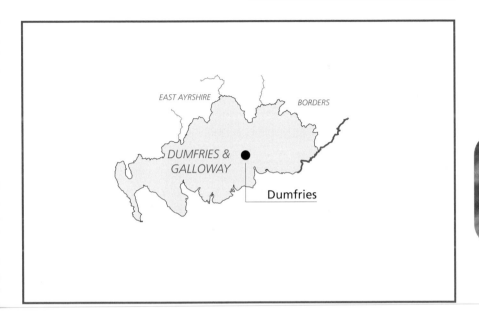

Complementary therapy services in

Dumfries & Galloway

Dumfries   • Dumfries & Galloway Cancer Support Group

Dumfries & Galloway Cancer Support Group

Susan Hayes or Pauline Mason **01387 711086 or 01387 267705**
Auchenleys, Kirkmahoe, Dumfries, Dumfries & Galloway DG1 1RE

Every month, group meetings are held in Dumfries at 1 Cresswell Gardens, off Barrie Avenue, every second and fourth Wednesday evening (19.00-21.30)

Therapies:	Art Therapy, Counselling, Massage, Meditation, Reiki, Relaxation, Visualisation
Details:	Available to clients and carers at group meetings through self referral. Advance booking is required
Cost:	All free of charge
	Fee for 'out of group' session in Massage and Reiki
Quality assurance:	Discussed before treatment
Promotion:	Leaflets and posters via hospitals, doctors, nurses, community health council, library, etc

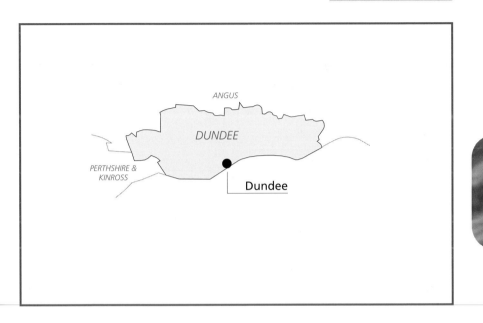

Complementary therapy services in

Dundee

Dundee   • NHS Tayside

NHS Tayside

Liz Goss, Service Manager   **01382 423137**

Roxburghe House, Royal Victoria Hospital, Jedburgh Road, Dundee DD2 1SP

Therapies:	Acupuncture, Aromatherapy, Art Therapy, Reflexology, Reiki, Relaxation
Details:	Availability of service varies
To clients:	All therapies are available to clients with Aromatherapy, Reflexology, Reiki and Relaxation also open to staff. Aromatherapy, Art Therapy, Reflexology, Reiki and Relaxation through professional referral
Cost:	All free of charge
Quality assurance:	All potential clients are patients within our service and are referred by a keyworker

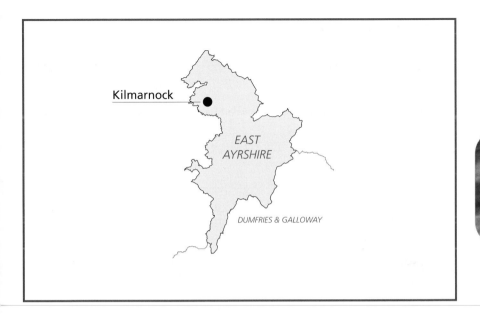

Complementary therapy services in

East Ayrshire

Kilmarnock   • Ayrshire Cancer Support

Ayrshire Cancer Support

Irene Wilson RGN, Dip Couns Dip Ca Nursing   **01563 538008**

16 Portland Road, Kilmarnock, East Ayrshire KA1 2BS

Therapies:	Aromatherapy, Art Therapy, Hypnotherapy/Hypnosis, Reflexology, Reiki, Relaxation
Details:	All therapies are available to clients and carers on weekdays through self referral, with Relaxation also open to staff. Advance booking is required
Cost:	All free of charge
Quality assurance:	GP or consultant's permission is obtained. For Hypnotherapy/Hypnosis, Aromatherapy and Reflexology, all carried out by fully trained therapists
Materials supplied:	Information on specific therapies given to clients
Promotion:	Leaflets and posters. Liaison with health professionals in acute trusts, primary care trusts and local hospice. Local media. Website (www.ayrshirecancersupport.org)

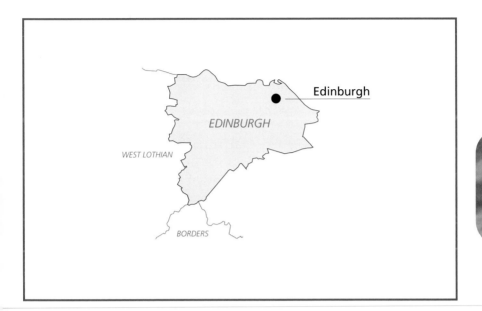

Complementary therapy services in

Edinburgh

| Edinburgh | • Edinbugh Royal Infirmary |
| | • Marie Curie Centre – Fairmile |

Edinbugh Royal Infirmary

Joan Adam, Clinical Nurse Specialist **0131 536 1735**
Palliative Care Service, 1 Lauriston Place, Edinburgh EH3 9YW

The complementary therapy service is directed at inpatients under the care of the palliative service

Therapies:	Aromatherapy, Massage
Details:	Available to clients and carers on weekday afternoons through professional referral (a voluntary service; please contact for details of availability)
Cost:	All free of charge
Quality assurance:	Patients are screened by the palliative care team. Allergies are checked by therapists. The massage and essential oils are very safe and gentle
Promotion:	Through a referral from the palliative care team

Marie Curie Cancer Care – Fairmile

Stephen Smith, Clinical Services Manager **0131 470 2201**
Frogston Road West, Edinburgh EH10 7DR

Therapies:	Aromatherapy, Massage, Relaxation, Visualisation
Details:	Available to clients on Tuesday mornings through professional referral
Cost:	All free of charge
Quality assurance:	Medical and nursing staff complete a screening form for each patient prior to receiving massage
Promotion:	Discussion with patients by members of staff following assessment

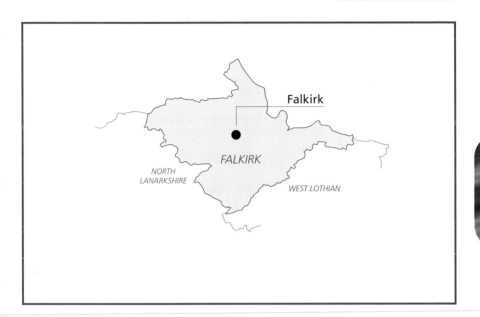

Complementary therapy services in

Falkirk

Falkirk • Forth Valley Acute Hospital NHS Trust

Forth Valley Acute Hospital NHS Trust

Liz MacMillan, Team Leader   **01324 624 200 x5772 (bleep 309)**
Oncology Nurse Team, Major's Loan, Falkirk FK1 5QE

Therapies:	Aromatherapy, Massage
Details:	Available to clients on professional referral. Advance booking required
Cost:	All free of charge
Quality assurance:	Strict medical history taken. Permission from GP or medical consultant is obtained
Promotion:	Word of mouth

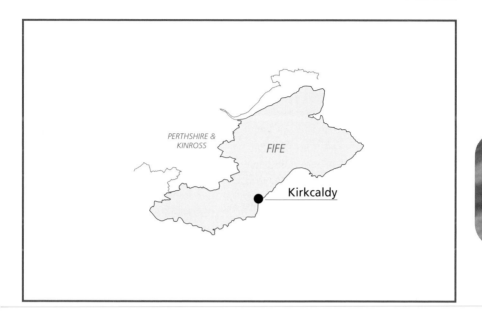

Complementary therapy services in

Fife

Kirkcaldy   • Victoria Hospice

Victoria Hospice

Jane Morris, Charge Nurse   **01592 648072**

Fife Acute Hospital NHS Trust, Victoria Hospital, Hayfield Road, Kirkcaldy, Fife KY2 5AH

The hospice is set in the grounds of Victoria Hospital and houses a 10-bed unit and 15 day places available Monday to Friday

Therapies:	Acupuncture, Aromatherapy, Art Therapy, Counselling, Massage, Nutritional Programmes, Reflexology, Relaxation, Nutritional Supplements, Visualisation
Details:	All therapies are available to clients on weekdays through self referral, with Counselling also open to carers. Advance booking and drop-in available
Cost:	All free of charge
Quality assurance:	All clients are assessed by medical staff prior to receiving complementary therapies. Written consent is obtained. Contra-indications are discussed with therapist and client. Nursing or medical staff refer to dietician who sees most clients as inpatients
Promotion:	Information leaflets about the hospice

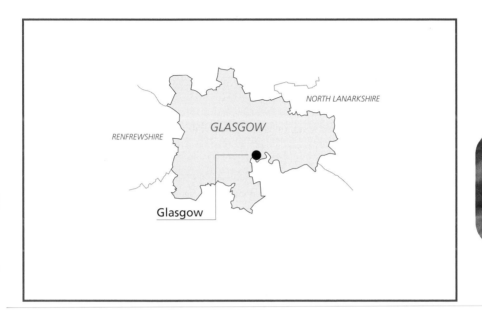

NORTH LANARKSHIRE

GLASGOW

RENFREWSHIRE

Glasgow

Complementary therapy services in

Glasgow

Glasgow
- Marie Curie Cancer Care
- Tak Tent Cancer Support Scotland

Marie Curie Cancer Care

Wilma Stewart, Day Services Manager   **0141 531 1332**
Marie Curie Centre, Hunter's Hill, 1 Belmont Road, Springburn, Glasgow G21 3AY

A specialist palliative care centre

Therapies:	Acupuncture, Aromatherapy, Art Therapy, Counselling, Massage, Reflexology, Reiki, Relaxation, Shiatsu, Spiritual Healing, Nutritional Supplements, Visualisation
Details:	All therapies are available to clients, carers and staff on weekdays (and Wednesday evenings) through professional referral. Drop-in for all complementary therapies or book in advance for all except Counselling
Cost:	All free of charge
Quality assurance:	Clinical nurse specialist makes initial assessment. Therapist then makes own assessment. Full history is available – if there is a doubt, patient can be medically assessed
Materials supplied:	Leaflets; relaxation tapes given to patients and carers
Promotion:	Leaflets; in-house education programme

Tak Tent Cancer Support Scotland

Mrs Carol Horne, Manager   **0141 2110122**
Flat 5, 30 Shelley Court, Gartnavel Complex, Glasgow G12 0YN

Voluntary organisation providing support to people affected by cancer

Therapies:	Aromatherapy, Massage, Reflexology, Reiki
Details:	Available to clients, carers and staff on Monday mornings, Tuesdays and Fridays (evenings if clients request appointments) through self referral although clients must have clinicians' consent if disease is active. Advance booking required

Cost: All free of charge

Quality assurance: Therapists take confidential case history. Clinicians' permission
                        sought by patients. Booking process ascertains status of client
                        and links to appropriate therapists

Materials supplied: General leaflet from organisation and information sheets on
                        therapies from therapists

Promotion: Leaflets; posters; word of mouth; website

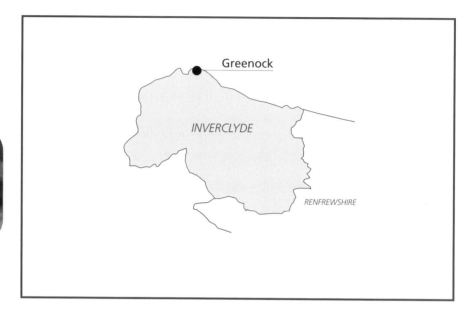

Complementary therapy services in

Inverclyde

Greenock   •   Ardgowan Cancer Care Education & Support Service

Ardgowan Cancer Care Education & Support Service

Leigh Murray   **01475 558855**

Ardgowan Hospice, 12 Nelson Street, Greenock, Inverclyde PA15 1TS

A cancer resource centre offering outpatient services and a drop-in facility from the moment of diagnosis

Therapies:	Aromatherapy, Massage, Reflexology, Reiki, Relaxation, Visualisation
Details:	All therapies are available through self referral to clients on weekdays (including Wednesday evening); availability varies from week to week. Aromatherapy, Massage, Reflexology and Reiki also open to carers. Book in advance for Aromatherapy, Massage, Reflexology and Reiki; drop-in for Relaxation and Visualisation
Cost:	All free of charge
Quality assurance:	Policy and procedures. Client assessment, including medical history. Discussion with other health professionals. Corresponding with GP/oncology team if there are any doubts
Materials supplied:	CancerBACUP, own leaflets, videos, etc
Promotion:	Promotional materials – leaflets, posters, business cards; awareness events – medical faculty, nurses, public; newspaper articles and advertisements; word of mouth; Macmillan nursing team and other health professionals

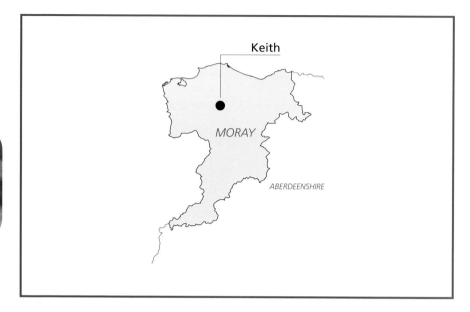

Complementary therapy services in

Moray

Keith   • Keith Cancer Link

Keith Cancer Link

Adeline Reid, Chairman   **01542 881008**
Health Centre, Turner Street, Keith, Moray AB55 5DJ

Located in the town centre, with easy access for the disabled. Meetings are held on the ground floor which is spacious, bright, comfortable and offers an excellent ambience for the group. Relaxation room and kitchen available

Therapies:	Aromatherapy, Art Therapy, Colour Therapy, Counselling, Crystal Therapy, Herbal Remedies, Hypnotherapy/Hypnosis, Massage, Indian Head (& Neck) Massage, Meditation, Music Therapy, Reflexology, Reiki, Relaxation, Shiatsu, Spiritual Healing, Therapeutic Touch, Visualisation
Details:	Available to clients and carers all week (including evenings) through self referral, with Reflexology also available to staff. Drop-in for Meditation, Relaxation and Visualisation; book in advance for Aromatherapy, Art Therapy, Counselling, Herbal Remedies, Hypnotherapy/Hypnosis, Massage, Music Therapy, Reflexology, Reiki, Shiatsu, Spiritual Healing and Therapeutic Touch
Cost:	All free of charge
Quality assurance:	All therapists are professionals. Audit carried out twice a year within group to gauge success of therapies. Full medical history taken on assessment. Patients/carers/families advised to inform patient's GP of any treatments being considered. Health clinic in town provides therapies. Transport provided to health clinic. Escort also provided if required
Materials supplied:	Cassettes, library, leaflets and information given routinely at meetings
Promotion:	Posters; media/local radio broadcasts/regular press reports; word of mouth; in the course of work as distict nurse; postcard for group information, which is also distributed to clinics

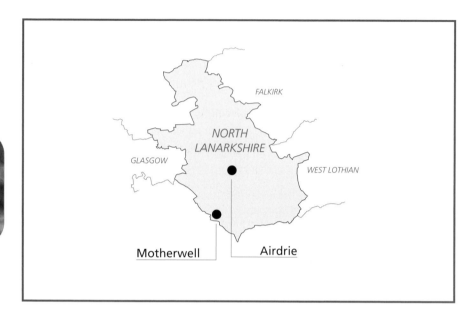

Complementary therapy services in

North Lanarkshire

Airdrie
- Monklands Hospital

Motherwell
- Dalziel Day Unit Hospice

Monklands Hospital

Patricia McCabe, Complementary Therapist   **01236 712419**
Monkscourt Avenue, Airdrie, North Lanarkshire ML6 0JS

A haematology/oncology ward with 10 inpatient beds and a busy day unit

Therapies:	Aromatherapy, Massage, Reflexology, Relaxation, Therapeutic Touch, Visualisation
Details:	All therapies are available to clients on weekdays, with Aromatherapy, Massage, Reflexology and Therapeutic Touch also open to carers and staff. Check with Monklands Hospital for referrals and availability
Cost:	All free of charge
Quality assurance:	Full consultation prior to any of the therapies. Colourful leaflets explaining all therapies available
Materials supplied:	Relaxation tapes, various literature
Promotion:	Leaflets; referrals from patient's consultant; referrals from GPs/Macmillan nurse specialist/palliative care nurse specialist

Dalziel Day Unit Hospice

Carol Murphy, Macmillan Nurse   **01698 245026**
Strathclyde Hosptal, Airbles Road, Motherwell, North Lanarkshire ML1 3BW

Care for the elderly in beautiful grounds

Therapies:	Acupuncture, Aromatherapy, Counselling
Details:	All therapies are available to clients on Monday afternoons through professional referral, with Counselling also available to carers. Advance booking is required
Cost:	All free of charge
Quality assurance:	Information given before treatment
Promotion:	Information leaflet

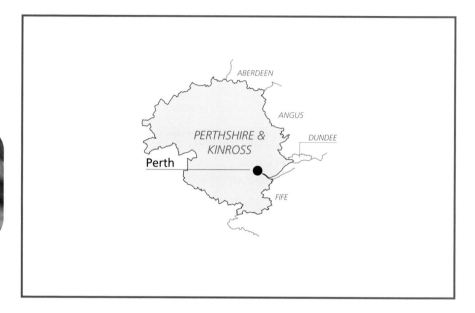

Complementary therapy services in
Perthshire and Kinross

Perth
- Macmillan House

Macmillan House

Ann Gourlay   **01738 639303**
Isla Road, Perth, Perthshire & Kinross PH2 7HQ

Therapies:	Aromatherapy, Art Therapy, Reflexology, Relaxation, Visualisation
Details:	All therapies are available to clients on Monday mornings, Tuesdays, Wednesday afternoons and Friday afternoons through both self and professional referral. Aromatherapy is also available to staff
Cost:	All free of charge Fee charged to staff for Aromatherapy
Quality assurance:	Therapist receives information on patient's condition
Promotion:	Information leaflet

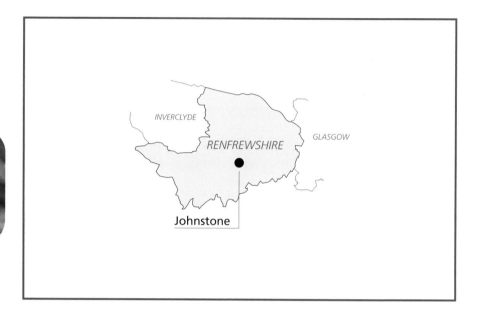

Complementary therapy services in

Renfrewshire

Johnstone   • St Vincent's Hospice

St Vincent's Hospice

Trudy Lafferty, Matron   **01505 705635**
Midton Road, Howwood, Johnstone, Renfrewshire PA9 1AF

Offers an 8-bedded inpatient unit, a day hospice which is available five days a week,
bereavement counselling, home respite and a home care service

Therapies:	Aromatherapy, Homeopathy, Massage, Reflexology, Reiki, Relaxation
Details:	All therapies are available on Monday afternoons, Tuesday afternoons, Wednesdays, Thursdays, and Friday mornings through professional referral. Aromatherapy, Massage, Reflexology, Reiki and Relaxation are also open to carers and staff. Advance booking is required
Cost:	All free of charge
Quality assurance:	Consent of medical staff obtained
Promotion:	Through patients already using the service; occasional referrals from our home care team

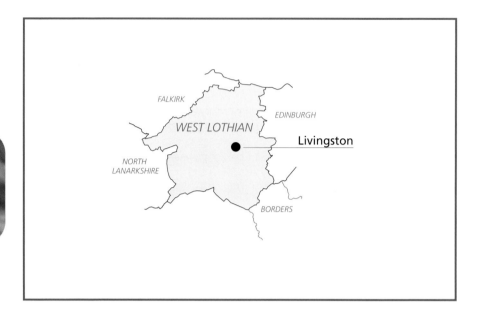

Complementary therapy services in
West Lothian

Livingston   • St John's Hospital at Howden

St John's Hospital at Howden

Brenda Bottrill   **01506 422753**
Howden Road West, Livingston, West Lothian EH54 6PP

Although attached to the main hospital, the facility has its own porch entrance and
conservatory to allow patients direct entry

Therapies:	Aromatherapy, Art Therapy, Counselling, Massage, Relaxation, Visualisation
Details:	Available to clients on weekdays (except Wednesdays) through self referral. Aromatherapy, Counselling, Massage, Relaxation and Visualisation are open to carers. Book in advance for Relaxation and Visualisation therapy (can be referred by healthcare professional); drop-in for Counselling, Relaxation and Visualisation
Cost:	Please enquire
Quality assurance:	The complementary therapist has many years' experience working with cancer patients and is very aware of disease process, stage of disease, etc. Through information from staff prior to treating a patient/carer
Materials supplied:	Cassettes
Promotion:	Included in information pack about unit; posters/leaflets

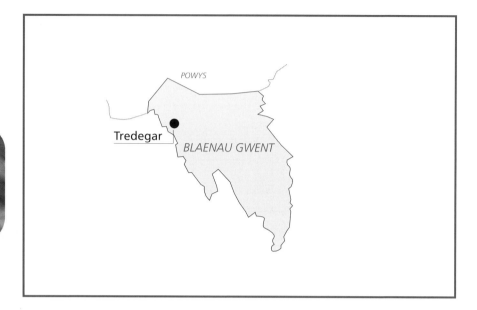

Complementary therapy services in

Blaenau Gwent

Tredegar   ● Hospice of the Valleys

Hospice of the Valleys

Dr Richard Lamerton, Medical Director   **01495 717277 or 07970 818498**
Hospice of the Valleys, Park Gates Business Centre, Morgan Street, Tredegar, Blaenau
Gwent NP22 3ND

From diagnosis onwards, the hospice offers: 24-hour on-call; hospice-at-home; weekly
drop-in; and monthly day clinics. It also operates drop-in centres in Abertillery and
Ebbw Vale, and plans the same for Brynmawr and Abergavenny

Therapies:	Acupuncture, Aromatherapy, Art Therapy, Qi Gong (Chi Kung), Counselling, Dream Therapy, Massage, Indian Head (& Neck) Massage, Thai Massage, Meditation, Nutritional Programmes, Reflexology, Relaxation, Shiatsu, Spiritual Healing, Visualisation, Yoga
Details:	All therapies are available to clients and carers through self referral (contact for availability), with Dream Therapy, Massage, Meditation and Spiritual Healing therapies open to staff. Drop-in for Massage, Nutritional Programmes, Reflexology, Relaxation, Spiritual Healing and Visualisation; all complementary therapies can be advance booked. Clients or carers may be referred by health professionals. Drop-in service available weekly for half a day in each town. Bookings are for the full-day clinic which is held twice a month
Cost:	All free of charge. We sometimes offer Reiki; our therapies are free of charge but we welcome donations
Quality assurance:	Patients' programmes prepared by whole team led by doctor. Patients are asked what therapies they would like and discuss their proposals with therapist. Therapists always warn patients of possible side effects
Materials supplied:	Library of books, videos and cassettes; leaflets on diet, dyspnoea, insomnia, chemotherapy and radiotherapy, etc
Promotion:	Articles in local papers; posters in GPs' surgeries and hospital outpatient departments; word of mouth

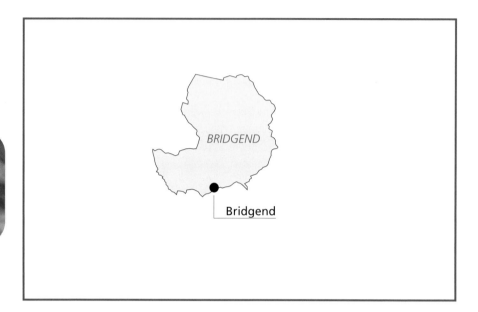

Complementary therapy services in

Bridgend

Bridgend
- Sandville Foundation
- Y Bwthyn Newydd

Sandville Foundation

Gwyneth Poacher, Nursing Director/Manager　　　　　**01656 743344**
Sandville Self-Help Centre, Sandville Court, Ton Kenfig, Bridgend CF33 4PT

The Sandville Foundation is situated in a large house with a therapy complex which includes a pool and offers 11 beds for overnight stays

Therapies:	Aromatherapy, Counselling, Herbal Remedies, Hypnotherapy/Hypnosis, Massage, Reflexology, Reiki, Relaxation, Spiritual Healing, Nutritional Supplements
Details:	Available to clients, carers and staff every day (10.00-16.00, including weekends, evenings if required) on self referral. Drop-in is available
Cost:	All free of charge
Quality assurance:	Yes
Promotion:	Leaflets; programmes

Y Bwthyn Newydd

Dr Rhian Owen　　　　　**01656 752014**
Princess of Wales Hospital, Coity Road, Bridgend CF31 1RQ

A specialist palliative service unit in the grounds of a District General Hospital. It comprises inpatients, day care and a base for hospital and community teams

Therapies:	Acupuncture, Art Therapy, Massage, Relaxation
Details:	Available to clients Monday to Thursday on professional referral. Advance booking is required
Cost:	All free of charge
Quality assurance:	Assessing nurse and doctor are appropriately qualified in complementary therapies
Materials supplied:	Cassettes for relaxation; CancerBACUP books on complementary therapies are available if required
Promotion:	Service information booklet; advised by team members

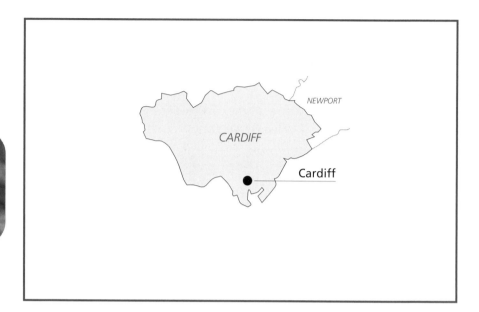

Complementary therapy services in

Cardiff

Cardiff
- George Thomas Hospice Care
- University Hospital of Wales
- Velindre NHS Trust

George Thomas Hospice Care

Chris Lloyd-Richards, Nurse Manager   **029 204 85345**
10 Tygwyn Road, Penylan, Cardiff CF23 5JE

Therapies:	Aromatherapy, Counselling, Massage, Reflexology, Relaxation
Details:	Available to clients and carers on professional referral. Operates Tuesdays, Wednesdays, Thursday afternoons and Fridays on both drop-in and advance bookings
Cost:	All free of charge
Quality assurance:	Assessment carried out. Agreement from GP
Materials supplied:	Provide tapes with relaxing music
Promotion:	Contact with nurses; centre leaflet

University Hospital of Wales

Mrs S Morgan   **029 20743377**
Palliative Care Team, Heath Park, Cardiff CF4 4XW

A hospital support team in the outpatient clinic

Therapies:	Acupuncture
Details:	Available to clients on weekday mornings through professional referral
Cost:	All free of charge
Quality assurance:	Assessed by consultant who is an acupuncturist

Velindre NHS Trust

Mrs Margaret Buckley-Harris   **029 20316925 x6945**

Velindre Road, Whitchurch, Cardiff CF14 2TL

Part of one of the largest oncology centres in the UK

Therapies:	Aromatherapy, Counselling, Reflexology, Relaxation, Nutritional Supplements
Details:	All therapies are available to clients with Counselling also open to carers. Reflexology is at no set time but on average four mornings a week. Relaxation one session a week for 6-8 weeks. Professional referral is required for Nutritional Supplements; self referrals accepted for Aromatherapy, Counselling, Reflexology and Relaxation. Advance booking is required for Reflexology and Relaxation
Cost:	All free of charge
Quality assurance:	Reflexology given only after a full assessment and the agreement of an oncologist
Promotion:	Staff make clients aware of Relaxation and Reflexology

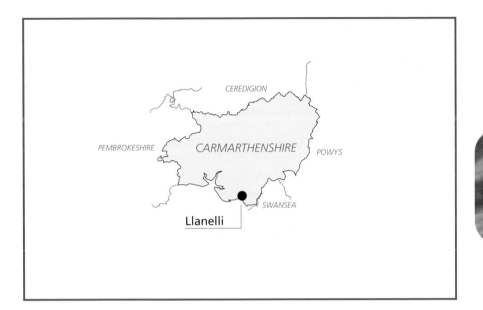

Llanelli

Complementary therapy services in
Carmarthenshire

Llanelli • Ty Bryngwyn Palliative Care Unit

Ty Bryngwyn Palliative Care Unit

Sister Mandy James   **01554 783563**
Ty Bryngwyn, Prince Philip Hospital, Llanelli, Carmarthenshire SA14 8QF

Based within hospital grounds, Ty Bryngwyn is a separate palliative care unit

Therapies:	Acupuncture, Counselling, Nutritional Programmes, Reflexology, Reiki, Relaxation, Nutritional Supplements
Details:	Acupuncture, Nutritional Programmes, Reflexology, Reiki, Relaxation and Nutritional Supplements therapies are available to clients; Counselling, Reflexology and Reiki to carers; and Acupuncture, Reflexology and Reiki to staff. Therapies are available on Tuesdays, Wednesday mornings and Thursdays. Professional referral is required for Reflexology; self referral accepted for Counselling, Nutritional Programmes, Reiki, Relaxation and Nutritional Supplements. Book in advance for Counselling (can be referred by a healthcare professional)
Cost:	All free of charge
Materials supplied:	Leaflets; promotion

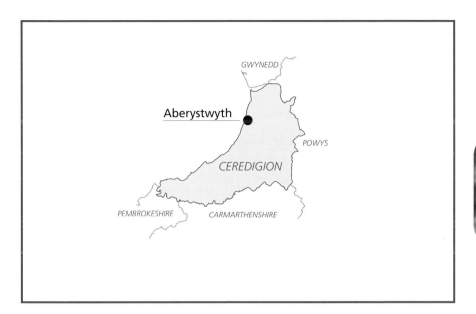

Complementary therapy services in

Ceredigion

Aberystwyth   • Bronglais Hospital

Bronglais Hospital

Nest Howells, Oncology Nurse   **01970 635752**
Ceredigtion, Aberystwyth, Ceredigion SY23 1ER

Bronglais is a medical ward with oncology beds and palliative care beds

Therapies:	Acupuncture, Aromatherapy, Art Therapy, Counselling, Massage, Reflexology, Reiki, Relaxation, Visualisation
Details:	All therapies are available to clients with Art Therapy, Counselling and Reiki open to carers, and Aromatherapy, Massage, Reflexology and Relaxation open to staff. Self referrals are accepted for Aromatherapy, Art Therapy, Counselling, Massage, Reflexology, Reiki, Relaxation and Visualisation; professional referral is required for Acupuncture. All therapies are available via advance booking but Aromatherapy, Art Therapy and Massage are also available on drop-in. Availability is negotiable; at present the service is limited as therapists are employed in another capacity (e.g. as nurses and occupational therapists)
Cost:	Please enquire
Quality assurance:	Policy in place. Staff are oncology trained or experienced health professionals
Materials supplied:	Tapes and literature, eg. about Bristol Cancer Help Centre
Promotion:	Drop-in centre monthly for patients and carers; verbal; leaflets

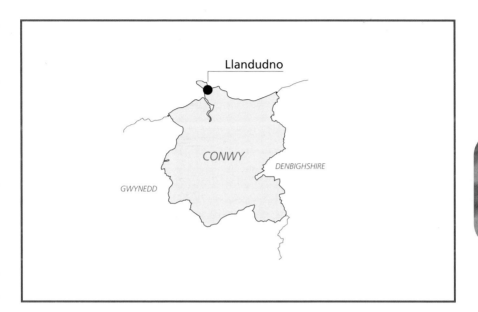

Complementary therapy services in
Conwy

Llandudno
- North Wales Holistic Cancer Care
- St David's Hospice

North Wales Holistic Cancer Care

Mrs Jean Tideswell, Chairperson　　　　　　　　　**01492 871984**

Jean's Health, Fitness and Natural Therapy Studio, 6 Garage Street, Llandudno, Conwy LL30 1DW

As well as the studio, the facility uses rooms at the community hospital, Hesketh Road, Colwyn Bay

Therapies:	Aromatherapy, Counselling, Massage, Meditation, Reflexology, Reiki, Relaxation, Spiritual Healing, Visualisation
Details:	All therapies are available to clients and carers on self referral. Therapies are available first and third Mondays in Llandudno and first and third Thursdays in Colwyn Bay. Advance booking is required
Cost:	Our therapies are free, but donations are welcomed
Quality assurance:	Patients, not carers, need letter of authorisation from GP/consultant for treatments/therapies. Full holistic assessment. Self-evaluation sheet
Materials supplied:	Audio cassettes
Promotion:	Posters; leaflets; press; word of mouth; referrals through information given by professionals

St David's Hospice

Mrs Irene Roberts, Senior Nurse　　　　　　　　　**01492 879058**

Abbey Road, Llandudno, Conwy LL30 2EN

The Hospice is located in a new, purpose-built building. Both the day care (opened September 1999) and inpatient (opened mid 2001) services cater for 10 places each

Therapies:	Aromatherapy, Art Therapy, Reflexology, Reiki, Visualisation
Details:	All therapies are available to clients, with Aromatherapy, Reflexology and Visualisation also open to carers, and

Aromatherapy and Reiki open to staff. Sessions run on
weekdays and are open to both professional (Aromatherapy)
and self referrals (Art Therapy). Aromatherapy is open to
drop-in

Cost:	All free of charge
Materials supplied:	Printed literature
Promotion:	Leaflets; posters; word of mouth; information days

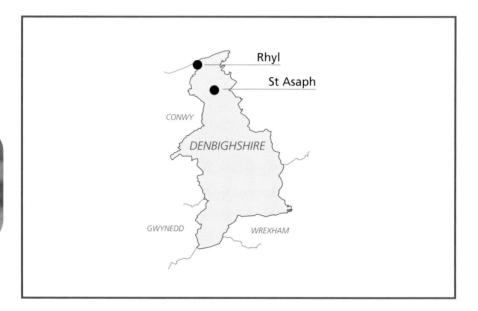

Complementary therapy services in

Denbighshire

Rhyl   ● North Wales Cancer Treatment Centre

St Asaph   ● St Kentigern Hospice and Palliative Care Centre

North Wales Cancer Treatment Centre

Clinical Nurse Manager   **01745 445150**
Rhuddlan Road, Bodelwyddan, Rhyl, Denbighshire LL18 5UL

The centre provides radiotherapy and chemotherapy facilities for people in North Wales. Gwynedd and Wrexham Hospitals provide chemotherapy services locally

Therapies:	Counselling, Massage, Relaxation
Details:	All therapies are available to clients, with Counselling and Relaxation also open to carers, and Counselling available to staff. Professional referral is required for Massage and Relaxation; self referrals accepted for Counselling. Therapies are available on Tuesdays, Thursday afternoons, Wednesday mornings (Massage) and Thursday evenings (Counselling). Availability of other therapies is in response to referrals. Advance booking is required
Cost:	All free of charge
Quality assurance:	Individuals are assessed initially by relevant therapist regarding suitability
Promotion:	Word of mouth; nurse/healthcare professionals

St Kentigern Hospice and Palliative Care Centre

Mrs Sam Tattersall, Matron/Manager   **01745 585221**
Upper Denbigh Road, St Asaph, Denbighshire LL17 0RS

Therapies:	Aromatherapy, Art Therapy, Massage, Reflexology, Reiki, Relaxation, Nutritional Supplements, Visualisation
Details:	Available through self referral to clients on weekdays except Monday afternoons. Book in advance for Aromatherapy, Massage, Reflexology, Reiki, Relaxation, Nutritional Supplements and Visualisation
Cost:	All free of charge

WALES Denbighshire

Quality assurance: All self-referred clients wanting Aromatherapy, Massage or Reflexology need permission from oncologist. The Centre has access to medical information; client is assessed; detailed, written records of the therapy undertaken and the evaluation of the treatment are kept

Materials supplied: Cassettes for Relaxation

Promotion: Posters; leaflets; verbal communications with other healthcare professionals

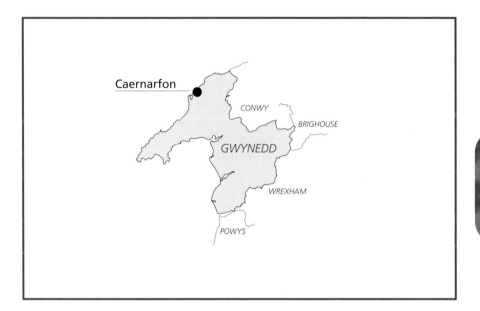

Complementary therapy services in

Gwynedd

Caernarfon   • Gwynedd Hospice at Home

Gwynedd Hospice at Home

Angela Jones, Macmillan Team Leader   **01286 662775**
Bodfan, Eryri Hospital, Caernarfon, Gwynedd LL55 2YE

Day care only is offered at the hospice

Therapies:	Aromatherapy, Reflexology, Reiki
Details:	Available to clients and carers on weekdays (except Wednesdays) through professional referral. Advance booking is required
Cost:	All free of charge
Quality assurance:	Complementary therapy policy includes: patient assessment documentation, GP agreement, therapists' qualification check
Promotion:	Through nursing service, clients and carers

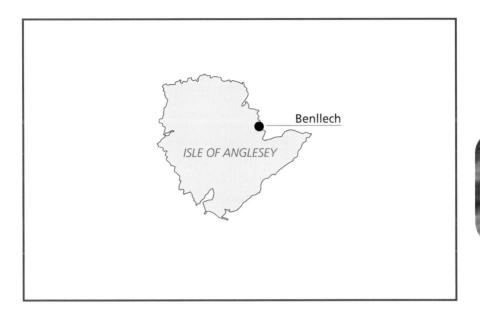

Benllech

ISLE OF ANGLESEY

Complementary therapy services in

Isle of Anglesey

Benllech

- Health Matters Benllech, Holistic Health Centre
  & Anglesey Breast Care

Health Matters Benllech, Holistic Health Centre & Anglesey Breast Care

Mrs Sheila Smith, Healthcare Consultant   **01248 852756 (Centre)**
or 490345 (Home)

3 Tryfan, Bangor Road, Benllech, Isle of Anglesey LL74 8TR

Located on the main road through Benllech with peaceful views out to sea. Anglesey is a peaceful island on which to recover!

Therapies: Acupuncture, Aromatherapy, Counselling, Herbal Remedies, Homeopathy, Meditation, Music Therapy, Nutritional Programmes, Relaxation, Shiatsu, Nutritional Supplements, Visualisation

Details: Available to clients, carers and staff on self referral. Sessions run on Thursdays, Fridays and Saturday mornings (contact for details of availability). Advance booking for Acupuncture, Aromatherapy, Counselling, Meditation, Music Therapy, Relaxation, Shiatsu and Visualisation; drop-in for Herbal Remedies, Homeopathy, Nutritional Programmes and Nutritional Supplements

Cost: There is a charge for Acupuncture, Aromatherapy, Counselling, Herbal Remedies, Homeopathy, Meditation, Music Therapy, Nutritional Programmes, Relaxation, Shiatsu, Nutritional Supplements, Visualisation

Materials supplied: Reference and lending library with over 1,000 books, videos and CDs; training

Promotion: Leaflets; posters locally; infrequent advertisements in local newspapers; hospital diary; networking

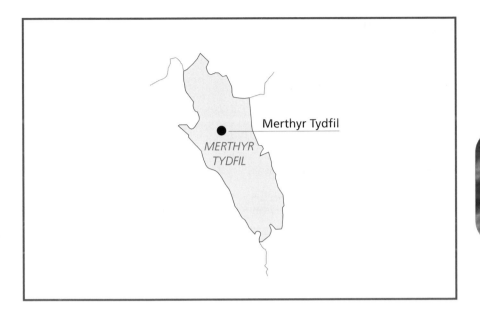

Complementary therapy services in

Merthyr Tydfil

Mountain Ash   • Cancer Care Society

Cancer Care Society

Andrew Penny, Centre Manager **01443 479369**
3a Oxford Street, Mountain Ash, Merthyr Tydfil CF45 3PG

Another centre runs at 61 Victoria Street, Dowlais, Merthyr Tydfil (Tel: 01685 379633)

Therapies:	Aromatherapy, Counselling, Massage, Reflexology
Details:	All therapies are available to clients and carers on weekdays through self referral. Advance booking is required
Cost:	All free of charge
Quality assurance:	Consent form from medical practitioner. Understanding of patient's condition. Assessment of client by practitioners/therapists
Materials supplied:	Leaflets and books
Promotion:	Leaflets; posters; press releases; web site (www.cancercaresoc.demon.co.uk); advertising

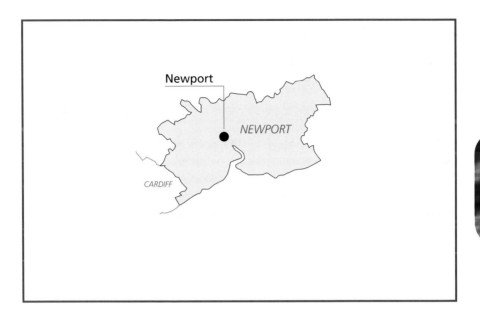

Complementary therapy services in

Newport

Newport ● St David's Foundation Hospice Care

St David's Foundation Hospice Care

Mr David Tapper   **01633 270980**

St David's Foundation, Cambrian House, St John's Road, Newport NP19 8GR

St David's is a community-based specialist palliative care service with two day hospices, a family support team, a hospice-at-home service, an education department and a complementary therapy service

Therapies:	Acupuncture, Aromatherapy, Massage, Reflexology, Reiki, Relaxation, Shiatsu, Visualisation
Details:	All therapies are by professional referral and are available to clients, with Aromatherapy, Massage, Reflexology, Reiki, Relaxation, Shiatsu and Visualisation also available to carers. Sessions run on weekdays (arrangements can be made for evening appointments). Advance booking is required
Cost:	All free of charge
Quality assurance:	All assessed by complementary therapist
Materials supplied:	Literature
Promotion:	Leaflets; posters; word of mouth; direct referral from primary healthcare teams and clinical nurse specialists

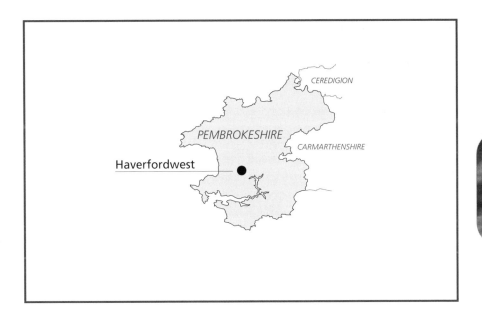

Complementary therapy services in

Pembrokeshire

Haverfordwest • Paul Sartori Foundation

Paul Sartori Foundation

Gillian Morse, Senior Clinical Nurse **01437 763223**

31 Haven Road, Haverfordwest, Pembrokeshire SA61 1DU

The Foundation is a hospice-at-home organisation

Therapies:	Aromatherapy
Details:	Available to clients and staff (availability depends on therapist) on both professional and self referral
Cost:	All free of charge
Quality assurance:	Even if client self-refers, we obtain referral form from health professional with extra information
Promotion:	Leaflets, talks to primary healthcare teams, hospitals, local groups

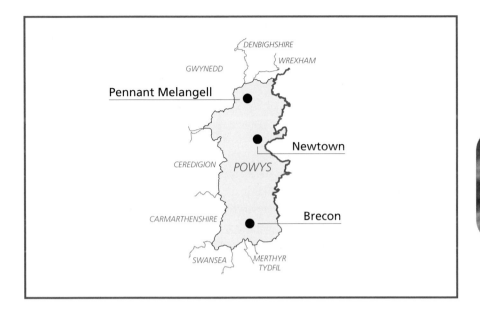

Complementary therapy services in

Powys

Brecon	● Usk House
Newtown	● Hafan Day Hospice
Pennant Melangell	● The Cancer Help Centre

Usk House

Sally Langworthy   **01874 611717**

Macmillan Service, Bridge Street, Llanfaes, Brecon, Powys LD3 0LU

Usk House runs a day hospice

Therapies:	Aromatherapy, Art Therapy, Counselling, Massage, Meditation, Relaxation, Therapeutic Touch
Details:	All therapies are available to clients and carers on self and professional referral (Counselling), with Counselling and Therapeutic Touch also available to staff. Sessions run on Monday mornings, Tuesdays, Wednesdays, and Friday mornings. Book in advance for Therapeutic Touch; drop-in available for Art Therapy, Meditation and Relaxation
Cost:	All free of charge
Quality assurance:	Most treatments are given after consultation with duty nurse
Promotion:	Leaflets; word of mouth

Hafan Day Hospice

Linda Jones, Palliative Care Sister   **01686 610215**

Newtown Hospital, Llanfair Road, Newtown, Powys SY16 2DW

A day hospice

Therapies:	Reflexology
Details:	Available to clients on Tuesdays and Wednesdays through professional referral. All complementary therapies are available via advance booking and drop-in
Cost:	All free of charge
Quality assurance:	Therapists are given full medical history
Promotion:	Leaflets; through GPs and other health professionals

The Cancer Help Centre

Judith Prust, Administrator　　　**01691 860408 (Tue – Fri from 10am to 4pm)**
The Melangell Centre, Pennant Melangell, Powys SY10 0HD

Located in a very rural area of Mid-Wales

Therapies:	Counselling
Details:	Available to clients, carers and staff from Tuesday to Friday (Wednesday evenings when necessary) on self referral. Advance booking is required
Cost:	Please enquire
Promotion:	Leaflets

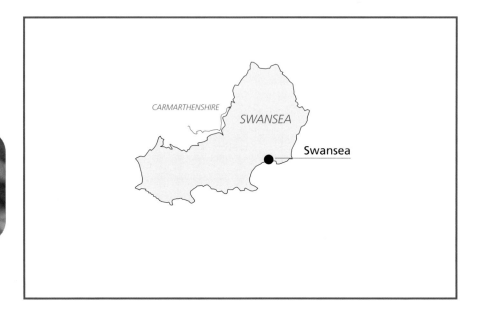

Complementary therapy services in

Swansea

Swansea
- Gower Cancer Self Help Group
- Morriston Hospital

Gower Cancer Self Help Group

Joy   **01792 203029**
Burrows Hall Nursing Home, Llangennith, Swansea SA3 1JB

Therapies: Aromatherapy, Art Therapy, Counselling, Homeopathy,
                     Massage, Meditation, Reflexology, Reiki, Relaxation, Spiritual
                     Healing, Therapeutic Touch, Visualisation
Details: Runs on Saturdays with all therapies available to clients on self
                     referral. Aromatherapy, Counselling, Massage, Meditation,
                     Reflexology, Relaxation and Visualisation are open to carers,
                     and Counselling, Meditation, Relaxation and Visualisation are
                     open to staff
Cost: All free of charge
Quality assurance: Consultation with client by trained therapists. Medication
                     taken into consideration before any therapy is undertaken.
                     Also have access to GP when necessary
Materials supplied: Via an in-house library
Promotion: Leaflets; posters; newspaper articles; word of mouth; hospital
                     displays

Morriston Hospital

Helen Walsh, Macmillan Senior Nurse   **01792 703412**
Palliative Care, Morriston, Swansea SA6 6NL

Therapies: Acupuncture, Relaxation
Details: Available to clients referred by a doctor
Cost: All free of charge
Promotion: Medical assessment that Acupuncture may be useful; part of
                     planned day care programme; individual patient assessment

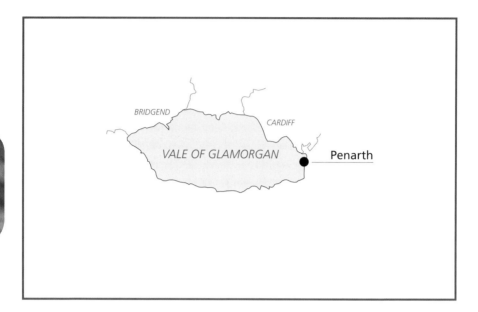

Complementary therapy services in

Vale of Glamorgan

Penarth   ● Marie Curie Cancer Care

Marie Curie Cancer Care

Andrew Wilson   **029 20426000**

Holme Tower, Bridgeman Road, Penarth, Vale of Glamorgan CF64 3YR

Provides a 30-bedded palliative care unit, day therapy and a community team

Therapies:	Acupuncture, Aromatherapy, Art Therapy, Drama Therapy, Massage, Music Therapy, Reflexology, Relaxation, Therapeutic Touch
Details:	All therapies are available to clients Monday to Thursday on professional referral, with Aromatherapy, Art Therapy, Drama Therapy, Massage, Music Therapy, Reflexology, Relaxation and Therapeutic Touch also open to carers. All complementary therapies can be booked in advance; drop-in available for Art Therapy, Drama Therapy, Music Therapy and Relaxation
Cost:	All free of charge
Quality assurance:	Assessment by each therapist
Promotion:	Leaflets, information given during assessment

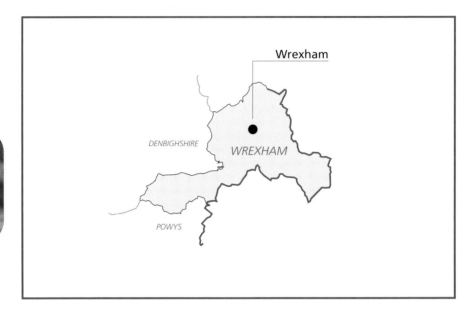

Complementary therapy services in

Wrexham

Wrexham
- Fight Cancer Together Club
- Nightingale House Hospice

Fight Cancer Together Club

Carolyn Roberts   **01691 772430**
Chirk Community Hospital, Chirk, Wrexham LL14 4AW

Therapies: Massage, Reflexology, Reiki, Relaxation, Visualisation
Details: Available to clients and carers on Wednesdays through self
                        referral
Cost: Please enquire
Quality assurance: In-depth assessment. Information on side effects. Information
                        booklets regarding patient's condition. Information on contra-
                        indications for treatment
Promotion: Leaflets; word of mouth

Nightingale House Hospice

Maralyn Joyce Land   **01978 316800**
Chester Road, Wrexham LL11 2SJ

Therapies: Acupuncture, Aromatherapy, Art Therapy, Bowen Technique,
                        Counselling, Massage, Reflexology, Relaxation
Details: All therapies are available to clients on weekdays through
                        professional referral, with Aromatherapy, Art Therapy, Bowen
                        Technique, Counselling, Massage, Reflexology and Relaxation
                        also open to carers, and Aromatherapy, Bowen Technique,
                        Counselling, Massage and Reflexology open to staff. Book in
                        advance for Bowen Technique
Cost: All free of charge
Quality assurance: Clinical assessments. Series of questions
Promotion: Leaflets; word of mouth; community nursing teams;
                        physiotherapists

Index 1

Availability of therapies across the country

Acupuncture

ENGLAND

Bedfordshire
Bristol
Cheshire
Derbyshire
Devon
Durham
East Sussex
Essex
Gloucestershire
Greater London
Greater Manchester
Hampshire
Herefordshire
Isle of Man
Isle of Wight
Kent
Merseyside
Norfolk
North Yorkshire
Northumberland
Nottinghamshire
Oxfordshire
Shropshire
Somerset
South Yorkshire
Suffolk
Surrey
Tyne & Wear
West Sussex
West Yorkshire
Worcestershire

NORTHERN IRELAND

Antrim

SCOTLAND

Angus
Dundee
Fife
Glasgow
North Lanarkshire

WALES

Blaenau Gwent
Bridgend
Cardiff
Carmarthenshire
Ceredigion
Gwynedd
Isle of Anglesey
Newport
Swansea
Vale of Glamorgan
Wrexham

Alexander Technique

ENGLAND

Devon
Greater London
Lancashire
Northumberland

Aromatherapy

ENGLAND

Bedfordshire
Berkshire
Bristol
Buckinghamshire
Cambridgeshire
Cheshire
Cornwall
Cumbria
Derbyshire
Devon
Dorset
Durham
East Sussex
East Yorkshire
Essex
Gloucestershire
Greater London
Greater Manchester
Hampshire
Herefordshire
Hertfordshire
Isle of Man
Isle of Wight
Kent
Lancashire
Leicestershire
Lincolnshire
Merseyside
Norfolk
North Yorkshire
Northamptonshire
Northumberland

Nottinghamshire
Oxfordshire
Shropshire
Somerset
South Yorkshire
Staffordshire
Suffolk
Surrey
Tyne & Wear
Warwickshire
West Midlands
West Sussex
West Yorkshire
Wiltshire
Worcestershire

NORTHERN IRELAND

Antrim
Derry

SCOTLAND

Aberdeenshire
Angus
Dundee
East Ayrshire
Edinburgh
Falkirk
Fife
Glasgow
Inverclyde
Moray
North Lanarkshire
Perthshire & Kinross
Renfrewshire
West Lothian

WALES

- Blaenau Gwent
- Bridgend
- Cardiff
- Carmarthenshire
- Ceredigion
- Conwy
- Denbighshire
- Gwynedd
- Isle of Anglesey
- Merthyr Tydfil
- Newport
- Pembrokeshire
- Powys
- Swansea
- Vale of Glamorgan
- Wrexham

Art Therapy

ENGLAND

- Bedfordshire
- Berkshire
- Bristol
- Cambridgeshire
- Cheshire
- Cornwall
- Cumbria
- Derbyshire
- Durham
- East Sussex
- East Yorkshire
- Essex
- Gloucestershire
- Greater London

- Greater Manchester
- Hampshire
- Hertfordshire
- Kent
- Lancashire
- Leicestershire
- Lincolnshire
- Merseyside
- Norfolk
- North Yorkshire
- Northamptonshire
- Northumberland
- Nottinghamshire
- Oxfordshire
- Shropshire
- South Yorkshire
- Staffordshire
- Suffolk
- Surrey
- Tyne & Wear
- Warwickshire
- West Midlands
- West Sussex
- West Yorkshire
- Wiltshire
- Worcestershire

NORTHERN IRELAND

- Antrim

SCOTLAND

- Aberdeenshire
- Angus
- Dumfries & Galloway
- Dundee

East Ayrshire
Fife
Glasgow City
Moray
Perthshire & Kinross
West Lothian

WALES

Blaenau Gwent
Bridgend
Ceredigion
Conwy
Denbighshire
Powys
Swansea
Vale of Glamorgan
Wrexham

Autogenic training

ENGLAND

Devon
Greater London

Bach Flower Remedies (or Flower Essences)

ENGLAND

Gloucestershire
Kent

Bowen Technique

ENGLAND

Worcestershire

WALES

Wrexham

Chiropractic

ENGLAND

Essex
Merseyside
Somerset
West Sussex

Colour Therapy

SCOTLAND

Moray

Counselling

ENGLAND

Bedfordshire
Berkshire
Bristol
Buckinghamshire
Cambridgeshire
Cheshire
Devon
Dorset
Durham

East Sussex
East Yorkshire
Essex
Gloucestershire
Greater London
Greater Manchester
Hampshire
Hertfordshire
Isle of Man
Isle of Wight
Kent
Lancashire
Leicestershire
Lincolnshire
Merseyside
North Yorkshire
Northumberland
Nottinghamshire
Oxfordshire
Shropshire
Somerset
South Yorkshire
Staffordshire
Suffolk
Surrey
Tyne & Wear
Warwickshire
West Midlands
West Sussex
West Yorkshire
Wiltshire
Worcestershire

NORTHERN IRELAND

Antrim
Derry

SCOTLAND

Aberdeenshire
Dumfries & Galloway
Fife
Glasgow
Moray
North Lanarkshire
West Lothian

WALES

Blaenau Gwent
Bridgend
Cardiff
Carmarthenshire
Ceredigion
Conwy
Denbighshire
Isle of Anglesey
Gwynedd
Merthyr Tydfil
Powys
Swansea
Wrexham

Cranio-Sacral Therapy

ENGLAND

Devon
Greater London
Greater Manchester

Kent
Merseyside

Crystal Therapy

SCOTLAND

Moray

Dance Therapy

ENGLAND

Norfolk

Drama Therapy

ENGLAND

Cambridgeshire
Greater London
Kent
Staffordshire
West Yorkshire
Wiltshire

WALES

Vale of Glamorgan

Dream therapy

WALES

Blaenau Gwent

Herbal Remedies

ENGLAND

Essex
Greater London
Lincolnshire
Merseyside
Norfolk
Surrey
West Sussex

NORTHERN IRELAND

Derry

SCOTLAND

Moray

WALES

Bridgend
Isle of Anglesey

Homeopathy

ENGLAND

Bristol
Devon
Essex
Greater London
Greater Manchester
Hertfordshire
Merseyside
Norfolk
Shropshire
South Yorkshire

Surrey
West Sussex
Worcestershire

NORTHERN IRELAND

Antrim
Derry

SCOTLAND

Renfrewshire

WALES

Isle of Anglesey
Swansea

Hypnotherapy/Hypnosis

ENGLAND

Berkshire
Cheshire
Derbyshire
East Yorkshire
Greater London
Kent
Lancashire
North Yorkshire
Surrey
Tyne and Wear

NORTHERN IRELAND

Antrim

SCOTLAND

Angus
East Ayrshire
Moray

WALES

Bridgend

Iscador

ENGLAND

Bristol
Greater London
Merseyside

Massage

ENGLAND

Bedfordshire
Berkshire
Bristol
Buckinghamshire
Cambridgeshire
Cheshire
Cornwall
Cumbria
Derbyshire
Devon
Dorset
Durham
East Sussex
East Yorkshire
Essex
Gloucestershire

Greater London

Greater Manchester

Hampshire

Herefordshire

Hertfordshire

Isle of Man

Isle of Wight

Kent

Lancashire

Leicestershire

Lincolnshire

Merseyside

Norfolk

North Yorkshire

Northamptonshire

Northumberland

Nottinghamshire

Oxfordshire

Shropshire

Somerset

South Yorkshire

Suffolk

Surrey

Tyne and Wear

Warwickshire

West Midlands

West Sussex

West Yorkshire

Wiltshire

Worcestershire

NORTHERN IRELAND

Antrim

Derry

SCOTLAND

Angus

Dumfries & Galloway

Edinburgh

Falkirk

Fife

Glasgow

Inverclyde

Moray

North Lanarkshire

Renfrewshire

West Lothian

WALES

Blaenau Gwent

Bridgend

Cardiff

Carmarthenshire

Ceredigion

Conwy

Denbighshire

Merthyr Tydfil

Newport

Powys

Swansea

Vale of Glamorgan

Wrexham

Massage – Bio-dynamic

ENGLAND

Greater London

Massage – Chair

ENGLAND

Greater Manchester

Massage – Indian Head (& Neck)

ENGLAND

Cumbria
Derbyshire
Devon
Hampshire
Hertfordshire
Kent
Leicestershire
Northumberland
Surrey
West Midlands
Worcestershire

SCOTLAND

Moray

WALES

Blaenau Gwent

Massage – Thai

WALES

Blaenau Gwent

Meditation

ENGLAND

Bedfordshire
Bristol
Buckinghamshire
Cambridgeshire
Cheshire
Cornwall
Devon
Dorset
Durham
East Sussex
Essex
Greater London
Greater Manchester
Hertfordshire
Isle of Man
Lancashire
Merseyside
Norfolk
Nottinghamshire
South Yorkshire
Suffolk
Surrey
Warwickshire
West Midlands
West Sussex
West Yorkshire

NORTHERN IRELAND

Antrim
Derry

SCOTLAND
- Dumfries & Galloway
- Moray

WALES
- Blaenau Gwent
- Conwy
- Gwynedd
- Isle of Anglesey
- Powys
- Swansea

Music Therapy

ENGLAND
- Bedfordshire
- Berkshire
- Bristol
- Cambridgeshire
- Cornwall
- Devon
- Durham
- East Sussex
- East Yorkshire
- Essex
- Greater London
- Greater Manchester
- Hertfordshire
- Kent
- Lancashire
- Merseyside
- Norfolk
- North Yorkshire
- Northamptonshire
- Northumberland

Nottinghamshire
Oxfordshire
Shropshire
Staffordshire
Surrey
Tyne and Wear
West Midlands
West Sussex
West Yorkshire
Wiltshire
Worcestershire

SCOTLAND
- Moray

WALES
- Isle of Anglesey
- Vale of Glamorgan

Naturopathy

ENGLAND
- Essex
- Norfolk
- West Sussex

Neuro-linguistic Programming

ENGLAND
- Lancashire
- North Yorkshire

Nutritional Programmes

ENGLAND

Bristol
Cambridgeshire
Devon
East Yorkshire
Essex
Greater London
Greater Manchester
Isle of Man
Merseyside
Norfolk
North Yorkshire
Northamptonshire
Surrey
Tyne and Wear
Warwickshire
West Sussex
West Yorkshire
Worcestershire

NORTHERN IRELAND

Derry

SCOTLAND

Fife

WALES

Blaenau Gwent
Carmarthenshire
Isle of Anglesey

Nutritional Supplements

ENGLAND

Berkshire
Bristol
Cambridgeshire
Cheshire
Cumbria
Devon
Durham
East Sussex
East Yorkshire
Essex
Gloucestershire
Greater London
Greater Manchester
Hampshire
Isle of Man
Lancashire
Lincolnshire
Merseyside
Norfolk
Northamptonshire
Northumberland
Shropshire
Somerset
South Yorkshire
Tyne and Wear
Warwickshire
West Midlands
West Sussex
West Yorkshire
Worcestershire

NORTHERN IRELAND

Antrim
Derry

SCOTLAND

Borders
Fife
Glasgow

WALES

Bridgend
Cardiff
Carmarthenshire
Denbighshire
Isle of Angelsey

Osteopathy

ENGLAND

Devon
Essex
Hertfordshire
Shropshire
West Sussex

Psychotherapy

ENGLAND

Lancashire

Qi Gong (Chi Kung)

WALES

Blaenau Gwent

Reflexology

ENGLAND

Bedfordshire
Berkshire
Bristol
Buckinghamshire
Cambridgeshire
Cheshire
Cornwall
Cumbria
Derbyshire
Devon
Dorset
Durham
East Sussex
East Yorkshire
Essex
Gloucestershire
Greater London
Greater Manchester
Hampshire
Herefordshire
Hertfordshire
Isle of Man
Isle of Wight
Kent
Lancashire
Leicestershire
Lincolnshire
Merseyside
Norfolk
North Yorkshire
Northamptonshire
Northumberland

Nottinghamshire
Oxfordshire
Shropshire
Somerset
South Yorkshire
Suffolk
Surrey
Tyne and Wear
Warwickshire
West Midlands
West Sussex
West Yorkshire
Wiltshire
Worcestershire

Cardiff
Carmarthenshire
Ceredigion
Conwy
Denbighshire
Gwynedd
Merthyr Tydfil
Newport
Powys
Swansea
Vale of Glamorgan
Wrexham

Reiki

NORTHERN IRELAND

Antrim
Derry

SCOTLAND

Aberdeenshire
Angus
Dundee
East Ayrshire
Fife
Glasgow
Inverclyde
Moray
North Lanarkshire
Perthshire & Kinross
Renfrewshire

WALES

Blaenau Gwent
Bridgend

ENGLAND

Bedfordshire
Buckinghamshire
Cambridgeshire
Cheshire
Cornwall
Cumbria
Derbyshire
Devon
Durham
East Sussex
East Yorkshire
Essex
Gloucestershire
Greater London
Greater Manchester
Hampshire
Hertfordshire
Kent
Lancashire

Leicestershire
Merseyside
Norfolk
North Yorkshire
Northamptonshire
Northumberland
Nottinghamshire
Shropshire
Somerset
South Yorkshire
Suffolk
Surrey
Tyne and Wear
Warwickshire
West Midlands
West Sussex
West Yorkshire
Worcestershire

NORTHERN IRELAND

Antrim
Derry

SCOTLAND

Aberdeenshire
Angus
Dumfries & Galloway
Dundee
East Ayrshire
Glasgow
Inverclyde
Moray
Renfrewshire

WALES

Bridgend
Carmarthenshire
Ceredigion
Conwy
Denbighshire
Gwynedd
Newport
Swansea
Wrexham

Relaxation

ENGLAND

Bedfordshire
Berkshire
Bristol
Buckinghamshire
Cambridgeshire
Cheshire
Cornwall
Cumbria
Derbyshire
Devon
Dorset
Durham
East Sussex
East Yorkshire
Essex
Gloucestershire
Greater London
Greater Manchester
Hampshire
Herefordshire
Hertfordshire

Isle of Man
Isle of Wight
Kent
Lancashire
Leicestershire
Lincolnshire
Merseyside
Norfolk
North Yorkshire
Northamptonshire
Northumberland
Nottinghamshire
Oxfordshire
Shropshire
Somerset
South Yorkshire
Staffordshire
Suffolk
Surrey
Tyne and Wear
Warwickshire
West Midlands
West Sussex
West Yorkshire
Wiltshire
Worcestershire

NORTHERN IRELAND

Antrim
Derry

SCOTLAND

Aberdeenshire
Angus
Borders

Dumfries & Galloway
Dundee
Edinburgh
East Ayrshire
Fife
Glasgow
Inverclyde
Moray
North Lanarkshire
Perthshire & Kinross
Renfrewshire
West Lothian

WALES

Blaenau Gwent
Bridgend
Cardiff
Carmarthenshire
Ceredigion
Conwy
Denbighshire
Isle of Angelsey
Merthyr Tydfil
Newport
Powys
Swansea
Vale of Glamorgan
Wrexham

Shiatsu

ENGLAND

Bedfordshire
Bristol
Cambridgeshire

Devon
East Sussex
Essex
Greater London
Greater Manchester
Hertfordshire
Kent
Merseyside
Northumberland
Nottinghamshire
Shropshire
South Yorkshire
Surrey
Tyne and Wear
West Sussex
West Yorkshire

SCOTLAND

Glasgow
Moray

WALES

Blaenau Gwent
Isle of Anglesey
Newport

Spiritual Healing

ENGLAND

Bedfordshire
Bristol
Buckinghamshire
Cambridgeshire
Cheshire

Cornwall
Cumbria
Devon
East Sussex
East Yorkshire
Essex
Gloucestershire
Greater London
Greater Manchester
Hertfordshire
Isle of Man
Kent
Lancashire
Merseyside
Norfolk
North Yorkshire
Nottinghamshire
Oxfordshire
Shropshire
Somerset
South Yorkshire
Surrey
West Midlands
West Sussex
West Yorkshire

NORTHERN IRELAND

Derry

SCOTLAND

Aberdeenshire
Glasgow
Moray

WALES

Blaenau Gwent
Bridgend
Conwy
Swansea

T'ai chi

ENGLAND

Cornwall

NORTHERN IRELAND

Antrim

Therapeutic Touch

ENGLAND

Bedfordshire
Buckinghamshire
Cheshire
Devon
East Sussex
Essex
Greater London
Greater Manchester
Isle of Wight
Kent
Lancashire
Merseyside
Norfolk
Northamptonshire
Nottinghamshire
Shropshire
Surrey

Tyne and Wear
West Midlands
West Sussex
West Yorkshire
Worcestershire

NORTHERN IRELAND

Antrim
Derry

SCOTLAND

Angus
Moray
North Lanarkshire

WALES

Powys
Swansea
Vale of Glamorgan

Visualisation

ENGLAND

Bedfordshire
Berkshire
Bristol
Buckinghamshire
Cambridgeshire
Cheshire
Cornwall
Cumbria
Derbyshire
Devon
Dorset

Durham
East Sussex
East Yorkshire
Essex
Greater London
Greater Manchester
Hampshire
Hertfordshire
Isle of Man
Isle of Wight
Kent
Lancashire
Leicestershire
Lincolnshire
Merseyside
Norfolk
North Yorkshire
Nottinghamshire
Shropshire
Somerset
South Yorkshire
Suffolk
Surrey
Tyne and Wear
West Midlands
West Sussex
West Yorkshire
Worcestershire

NORTHERN IRELAND

Antrim
Derry

SCOTLAND

Aberdeenshire

Dumfries & Galloway
Fife
Glasgow
Inverclyde
Moray
North Lanarkshire
Perthshire & Kinross
West Lothian

WALES

Blaenau Gwent
Ceredigion
Conwy
Denbighshire
Isle of Anglesey
Newport
Swansea
Wrexham

Yoga

ENGLAND

Dorset
Greater London
Isle of Wight
Lancashire
Nottinghamshire

NORTHERN IRELAND

Antrim

WALES

Blaenau Gwent

AVAILABILITY OF THERAPIES

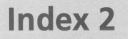

Index 2

Complementary
therapy services
listed by name

A

B

C

F

G

H

I

J

K

L

M

N

SERVICES LISTED BY NAME

O

P

Q

R

S

T

U

V

W

Y

Appendices

Appendix 1 – The Therapies

Descriptions abridged from the Encyclopedia of Natural Healing (Dorling Kindersley, 2000) by Anne Woodham and Dr David Peters with kind permission from the authors and the Penguin Group UK.

*Drama Therapy description kindly provided by Mezzi Franklin – drama therapist

Therapies	Description
Acupuncture	Part of Traditional Chinese Medicine, practitioners insert fine, sterile needles into specific points on the body as a treatment for disorders ranging from asthma to drug addiction. Acupuncture is increasingly practised in a simplified form by Western doctors; stimulation of acupoints can relieve nausea and help to alleviate pain.
Alexander Technique	Aims to improve posture so that the body can operate with minimum strain. By learning to stand and move correctly, stresses on the body are eased, and alleviating complaints that are exacerbated by poor posture allows all the body systems to function more efficiently.
Aromatherapy	Combining the medicinal properties known to exist in plants with the tradition of healing massage with oil. Molecules within the oils are said to enter through the bloodstream into the nervous system, influencing emotional and physical well-being. Aromatherapists employ many aromatic essential plant oils to treat physical and psychological conditions.
Art Therapy	Art therapy can help people in emotional distress, providing therapeutic relief in expression through creative activities such as painting, drawing and sculpting.
Autogenic Training	The therapy offers a rational, organised way to relax at will and mobilise the body's self-healing powers. It claims to alleviate

physical and mental problems, as well as improve work performance, creativity and personal relationships. It consists of a series of six mental exercises that allow the mind to calm itself by switching off the 'fight or flight' stress responses of the body.

Bach Flower Remedies (or Flower Essences)	Bach Flower Remedies are made by infusing or boiling plant material in spring water. Bach Flower Remedies and other flower essences are often taken for self-help during times of emotional crisis or stress.
Bowen Technique	This non-manipulative, hands-on technique is said to stimulate 'energy flow', enabling the body's self-healing resources to restore harmony. The practitioner makes a series of light rolling movements on the muscles and tendons. This is believed to encourage circulation, increase mobility and promote lymphatic drainage of waste products.
Chiropractic	Chiropractic seeks to diagnose and treat disorders of the spine, joints and muscles with techniques of manipulation, and to maintain the health of the central nervous system and organs.
Colour Therapy	The impact of colour on mood is widely recognised. Colour therapists go further, believing that different hues can treat illness and improve physical, emotional and spiritual health. Different colours are used to 'heal', often in the form of coloured light.
Counselling	Psychotherapy and counselling cover a wide range of techniques used to ease psychological suffering. Whether treating mental and emotional disorders or promoting self-awareness, these therapies offer the chance to understand and resolve difficult thoughts, feelings and situations by talking about them with a skilled listener.
Cranio-Sacral Therapy	A diagnostic and healing approach based on the application of corrective pressure to the cranium and sacrum. Cranio-Sacral therapy focuses on the membranes encasing the brain and spinal

	cord. Practitioners believe that it is these membranes that generate the cranial rhythmic impulse (CRI) of cerebrospinal fluid which affects the connective tissues linking all the organs, bones and muscles of the body. The aim of treatment is to ensure an even, rhythmic flow of CRI.
Crystal Therapy	Crystals, particularly quartz crystals such as amethyst and rose quartz, are believed to possess 'life energy', storing and discharging this rather like a battery. Practitioners often work by holding a crystal in one hand and resting the other on the part of your body which requires healing.
Dance Therapy	A method of expressing thoughts and feelings through movement. Participants are encouraged to move freely, sometimes to music. Dance therapy can be used to promote self-esteem and gain insight into emotional problems.
Drama Therapy *	The use of drama and narrative to explore emotions and gain insight into individual life experience which, in turn, will empower positive development.
Dream Therapy	Rapid eye movement (REM) sleep when most dreaming occurs, is thought to act as a psychological safety valve, helping us work through unconscious events and emotional issues. Practitioners recommend keeping a dream diary, jotting down details of a dream on waking, then analysing it for possible meaning.
Herbal Remedies	Diverse cultures use herbal remedies to treat disease and promote well-being. Many laboratory-produced drugs are derived from plants, but herbal remedies differ from conventional medicine in using parts of the whole plant rather than isolating single active ingredients.
Homeopathy	Homeopathy is a system of medicine based on the theory of 'like cures like' – a poison that causes symptoms of illness in a healthy

person can treat the same symptoms in someone who is ill. Substances are diluted many times to make a remedy that is safe to use, yet homeopaths believe sufficient 'likeness' remains between the remedy and the illness to stimulate the body's self-healing abilities.

Hypnotherapy/ Hypnosis	Practitioners induce a state of consciousness akin to deep daydreaming, in which the patient is deeply relaxed and open to suggestion, and can be desensitised to fears, phobias or pain.
Iscador	Iscador, an anthroposophical medicine extracted from mistletoe, can increase white blood cells (which fight infection) and affect the growth of cancer cells in the laboratory. (Anthroposophical medicine is a holistic approach to health following Rudolph Steiner's philosophy.)
Massage	Therapeutic massage can be used to promote general well-being and enhance self-esteem, whilst boosting the circulatory and immune systems to benefit blood pressure, circulation, muscle tone, digestion and skin tone. It has been incorporated into many health systems, and different massage techniques have been developed and integrated into various complementary therapies.
Massage Bio-dynamic	This form of massage aims to release energy believed to be bound up in the muscles and gut, causing physical and emotional pain. Discussion is encouraged, and techniques can be soothing and soporific, or more vigorous.
Massage Chair	As for massage – here the patient is massaged whilst sitting in a chair.
Massage Indian Head (& Neck)	This Ayurvedic head massage is said to relax the thin layer of muscle covering the head, improving blood flow, nourishing hair follicles and alleviating anxiety and stress. Practitioners

massage the shoulders and head with alternate firm and gentle strokes, using warm oil.

Massage Thai	Thai massage is a hybrid of the Chinese and Ayurvedic healing systems. The practitioner will use hands, feet and elbows to massage channels and points on the body through which prana, or 'vital force', is said to flow. Treatment involves a great deal of gentle stretching, bending and pulling, intended to restore or improve the flow of prana. It is also designed to induce a trance-like state that is believed to be psychologically beneficial.
Meditation	Meditation is intended to induce a state of profound relaxation, inner harmony and increased awareness. Various techniques can be used during meditation; all involve focusing the mind on a particular object or activity, and disregarding distractions.
Music Therapy	Making or responding to music can provide a real alternative to verbal communication, enabling the expression of emotions that may be too profound or primitive for words.
Naturopathy (Naturopathic Medicine)	Also known as 'natural medicine' or 'nature cure', naturopaths believe that the body's natural state is one of equilibrium, which can be disturbed by an unhealthy lifestyle. They look for the underlying causes of a problem rather than treating symptoms alone, combining diet and non-invasive therapies where possible to stimulate the healing process.
Neuro-linguistic Programming	Combining cognitive behavioural techniques with ideas from humanistic psychotherapy and from hypnotherapy. It works on the theory that life experiences, from birth onward, programme the way you see the world. You are taught consciously to change your patterns of speech and body language in order to communicate better and bring about personal change.

Nutritional Programmes/ Therapies	Embracing a wide range of approaches, nutrition-based complementary therapies seek to alleviate physical and psychological disorders through special diets and food supplements.
Nutritional Supplements	Believing that people can be nutritionally deficient even on a healthy diet, nutritional therapists prescribe vitamin and mineral supplements to treat a wide range of conditions.
Osteopathy	Practitioners use touch and manipulation of the musculo-skeletal system to restore or improve mobility and balance, and thereby enhance well-being. Techniques range from gentle massage to high-velocity mobilisation of the joints.
Psychotherapy	Psychotherapy and counselling cover a wide range of techniques used to ease psychological suffering. Whether treating mental and emotional disorders or promoting self-awareness, these therapies offer the chance to understand and resolve difficult thoughts, feelings and situations by talking about them with a skilled listener.
Qi Gong (Chi Kung)	Qi Gong translates literally as 'energy work'. A component element of Traditional Chinese Medicine, it is an ancient system of movement, breathing techniques and meditation, which is designed to develop and improve the circulation of qi or 'life energy', around the body. It is believed to help both body and mind to function at an optimum level, increasing vitality and encouraging self-healing mechanisms.
Reflexology	According to reflexologists, the feet and hands are a mirror of the body, and pressure placed on specific reflex points can be used to treat the corresponding areas of the body, in order to stimulate natural healing powers and promote well-being. All parts of the foot (or, less commonly, the hand) are massaged, so that the body as a whole is treated.

Reiki	A form of Japanese spiritual healing, practitioners draw on 'reiki energy', channelling it to areas of need in themselves and their patients.
Relaxation	Controlled breathing and the ability to relax at will are essential aspects of managing stress. Simple breathing exercises and muscle relaxation technique can be practised to reduce the physical and mental effects of stress, bringing therapeutic benefits such as lower heart rate, reduced blood pressure and lower levels of stress hormones.
Shiatsu	Shiatsu massage was developed in Japan. It has its basis in Traditional Chinese Medicine and follows the same principles of energy and meridians as acupressure – acupuncture without needles. The practitioner uses fingers, thumbs, elbows, knees and even feet in a combination of massage techniques, applying pressure to key points to influence and stimulate energy flow in the body.
Spiritual Healing	Healers describe their work as the 'restoration to health by non-physical means'; they channel benign healing energy to the patient to activate natural self-healing mechanisms. Spiritual healers regard themselves as conductors of healing forces.
T'ai Chi	This Chinese movement therapy is a non-combative martial art that uses breathing techniques and sequences of slow, graceful movements to improve the flow of qi, or 'life energy', calm the mind and promote self healing. T'ai Chi is often described as 'meditation in motion'. It is a dynamic form of Qi Gong.
Therapeutic Touch	Described as a modern form of the laying on of hands. Practitioners believe that the body has unique energy fields, defined in terms of quantum physics, and they use their hands to rebalance disruptions in the flow of energy and stimulate the patient's natural powers of self-healing.

Visualisation (Guided Imagery)	A technique that uses the imagination to help people cope with stress, fulfil their potential and activate the body's self-healing processes. Patients are said to be able to overcome physical and emotional problems by imagining positive images and desired outcomes to specific situations, either alone or helped by a practitioner (known as 'guided imagery').
Yoga	Best known in the West as a form of gentle exercise consisting of body postures and breathing techniques, yoga is in fact a complete system of mental and physical training. In the West it is valued more for its physical than spiritual benefits, such as its ability to increase suppleness and vitality, and to relieve stress.

Appendix 2 – Useful Resources

General Organisations

Macmillan Cancer Relief

UK Office, 89 Albert Embankment, London SE1 7UQ

Macmillan CancerLine: 0808 808 2020
Email: cancerline@macmillan.org.uk
Website: www.macmillan.org.uk

A UK charity that helps provide expert care and practical and emotional support for people living with cancer, including families, friends and carers. It funds specialist Macmillan nurses and doctors, builds vitally needed treatment centres, provides grants for patients with financial difficulties, offers training and resources to cancer self help and support groups and provides a range of information locally and nationally.

CancerBACUP

3 Bath Place, Rivington Street, London EC2A 3JR

Freephone help line: 0808 800 1234
Tel: 0207 696 9003 (general administration)
Email: info@cancerbacup.org
Website: www.cancerbacup.org.uk

Helps cancer patients, their families and friends live with cancer. Specialist cancer nurses provide information, practical advice and emotional support by telephone, letter and email. CancerBACUP produces a wide range of publications on all types of cancer and treatment. Local information centres operate in Nottingham, Coventry, Manchester, Kendal, Glasgow and London.

Marie Curie Cancer Care

89 Albert Embankment, London SE1 7TP

Tel: 020 7599 7777
Email: info@mariecurie.org.uk
Website: www.mariecurie.org.uk

Marie Curie is a national cancer care charity, providing practical hands-on nursing care at home and specialist multi-disciplinary care through Marie Curie centres. Both services are assessed through the local district nursing service and GPs/Consultants respectively. Both services are free of charge to cancer patients.

Tak Tent Cancer Support – Scotland
Flat 5, 30 Shelley Court, Gartnavel Complex, Glasgow G12 OYN

Tel:	0141 211 0122
Email:	tak.tent@care4free.net
Website:	www.taktent.org.uk

Support, information, counselling and complementary therapies for cancer patients, their relatives and friends. Network of groups meet throughout west and central Scotland, usually monthly, including one specifically for those aged 16-25 years.

Tenovus Cancer Information Centre
Velindre Hospital, Velindre Road, Whitchurch, Cardiff CF14 2TL

Freephone help line:	0808 808 1010
Tel:	02920 196 100
Email:	tcic@tenovus.com
Website:	www.tenovus.com

Provides psychological and practical support and information on all aspects of cancer for patients and their families. Services include: Freephone Cancer Helpline staffed by experienced cancer nurses; counsellors and social workers available for personal visits and one-to-one counselling; Oncology nurse specialists based at nine hospitals throughout Wales.

Ulster Cancer Foundation – Northern Ireland
40 – 42 Eglantine Avenue, Belfast BT9 6DX

Freephone help line:	0800 783 3339
Tel:	028 9066 3281
Email:	ucf.info@ulstercancer.org
Website:	www.ulstercancer.org

Provides a range of services for cancer patients and their families. These include a Freephone Cancer Helpline, staffed by cancer nurses; professional counselling; patient support groups; fitting service for women who have had breast surgery; headwear for those experiencing hair loss and a patient volunteer visiting service.

Complementary Therapy Organisations

Bristol Cancer Help Centre
Grove House, Cornwallis Grove, Clifton, Bristol BS8 4PG

Help line:	0117 980 9505
Tel:	0117 980 9500
Email:	info@bristolcancerhelp.org
Website:	www.bristolcancerhelp.org

Offers a healing programme that is complementary to medical treatment. It runs residential courses offering patients relaxation, meditation, visualisation, healing, counselling, nutritional advice, music and art therapy. Educational courses are also run for health professionals. Emotional support and information are available from the help line.

The Foundation for Integrated Medicine
12 Chillingworth Road, London N7 8QJ

Tel:	020 7619 6140
Fax:	020 7700 8434
Email:	enquiries@fimed.org
Website:	www.fimed.org

National charity promoting the integrated delivery of conventional and complementary medicine to make integrated healthcare available to all who need it. Information to healthcare professionals and the media; guidance for general public on finding a complementary therapy practitioner; newsletter and other publications about developments and good practice in integrated healthcare.

Research Council for Complementary Medicine
27a Devonshire Street, London W1N 1RJ

Email: info@rccm.org.uk
Website: www.rccm.org.uk

Founded in 1983, the Research Council for Complementary Medicine is a charity that aims to develop and extend the evidence base for complementary medicine in order to provide patients and practitioners with unequivocal statements of the effectiveness of individual therapies in the treatment of specific conditions. A database of research references and CAM Researcher Network can both be assessed on the website.

Books

Integrated Cancer Care - Holistic, complementary and creative approaches. Edited by Jennifer Barraclough. Oxford University Press, 2001. ISBN 0 19 263095 4

The Desktop Guide to Complementary and Alternative Medicine - an evidence-based approach. Edited by Edzard Ernst. Harcourt Publishers Ltd, 2001. ISBN 0 7234 3207 4

American Cancer Society's Guide to Complementary and Alternative Cancer Methods. American Cancer Society, 2000. ISBN 0-944235-24-7 (Available from www.amazon.com)

ABC of Complementary Medicine. Catherine Zollman and Andrew J. Vickers. BMJ Books, 2000. ISBN 0727912372

Encyclopedia of Natural Healing. Anne Woodham and Dr David Peters. Dorling Kindersley, 2000. ISBN 0 7513 1207 X

Booklets

Cancer and Complementary Therapies. CancerBACUP. (Freephone helpline: 0808 800 1234)

Reviews and reports

Complementary and Alternative Medicine – House of Lords Select Committee on Science and Technology, 2000. London: The Stationery Office.

Complementary therapies in cancer care - Abridged report of a study produced for Macmillan Cancer Relief. Kohn M, 1999.

Complementary Medicine - Information pack for primary care groups. NHS Executive, London in association with the Department of Health, Foundation for Integrated Medicine, NHS Alliance and National Association of Primary Care, 2000.

Integrated Healthcare: A Guide to Good Practice. Russo H. The Foundation for Integrated Medicine, 2000.

Professional organisation of complementary and alternative medicine in the United Kingdom. Mills S, Budd S. The Centre for Complementary Health Studies, University of Exeter, 2000.

Appendix 3 – How we compiled this directory

Macmillan Cancer Relief assembled a steering group to plan, manage and oversee the project. Its first task was to design a questionnaire for service providers to complete, and to compile a list of target recipients.

Contact lists were drawn up for the public and voluntary sectors using the following publications: The *2001 Directory of Hospice and Palliative Care Services in the United Kingdom and Republic of Ireland*[1] sponsored by Macmillan, Cancerlink's *Directory of Cancer Self Help and Support 2001/2*[2] and *Cancer Care 2000*[3] to identify NHS hospitals with cancer services.

In the case of hospital provision, we wrote to the lead cancer nurses or Macmillan specialist nurses in oncology, palliative care, haematology and paediatric departments. We felt these were the hospital departments most likely to have access to complementary therapies, or to provide them in-house.

Design of the questionnaire

Our questionnaire requested information on a wide range of issues. **Section A** sought details about basic provision for publication in this directory. We asked about the healthcare setting of the respondent (hospital, hospice etc), a description of it, and the geographical or catchment area served.

The questionnaire listed more than 20 therapies, to tick in the relevant boxes if any of them were provided. It requested details of any other therapy offered and asked if therapies were available just for cancer patients, or whether carers and staff could also take advantage of the services. We asked whether services were free or, if not, what the charge was. We also sought to find out how patients accessed the services; did they need a referral from a GP or a member of a medical or nursing team? Other questions asked about procedures to ensure treatment was safe and appropriate, and about the information/literature provided.

APPENDIX 3

Section B asked more detailed questions about attitudes to complementary therapies, and the professional training and accreditation of therapists. The information gathered in Section B was not intended for publication, but to help inform Macmillan policy-making in this area.

What therapies we included and why

We deliberated at length over which therapies to list in the questionnaire, as definitions, classifications and terminology continue to stir lively debate among health practitioners, academics and public alike.

The steering group consulted expert providers and reference texts in drawing up its list of therapies to feature on the questionnaire. They range from acupuncture and herbal therapies to meditation and art therapy. But some respondents gave us details of other therapies they were providing. A full list of the 42 therapies included in the directory, with a brief description of each one, appears in Appendix 1.

Inevitably, as the research base develops, and practices evolve to reflect the current body of evidence, some therapies once considered complementary have been integrated into conventional medical or nursing care. Acupuncture, for example, is now considered as mainstream in some quarters, commonly delivered by anaesthetists in pain clinics. Nevertheless, we judged that it merited inclusion in this directory.

We had various responses questioning the inclusion of counselling and creative therapies in our suggested list. However, since at least one of the reference texts (see Appendix 2), plus various expert opinions we consulted, supported their inclusion, we felt it reasonable to do so. We felt it important to be as inclusive as possible so that more patients have the option of accessing therapies that may help them now.

We have not judged the efficacy or effectiveness of individual therapies. If a therapy is classified as a complementary therapy by at least some reference texts and expert opinions, we have included it. For example, the Bowen technique and T'ai Chi are included on this basis.

Herbal and nutritional supplements used to complement orthodox care have been included. We recommend that patients wishing to take these should seek advice from their doctor because of possible adverse effects or interactions with other treatments. We have not, however, included alternative therapies intended to replace types of orthodox care, but only those intended to complement it.

Preliminary findings

From the replies received, we were able to capture sufficient data to feature 328 entries for the directory.

Our initial analysis of the responses to our questionnaire, and the methods we used to collect the information, has revealed the following:

- **Wide range of complementary therapies in use**

  We listed 20 therapies in our questionnaire – but providers told us of many more that were in use (see Appendix 1).

- **Cost and quality of complementary therapies varies**

  There is clearly no uniform policy on charging patients. Many services rely on NHS funding or financial support from the charitable and voluntary sector. Some providers raise money from the community to help meet their costs. Therapy sessions are often free of charge, although patient donations may be invited. Costs may be charged on a sliding scale, according to ability to pay.

  We asked respondents to give brief details of quality assurance policies underpinning their services. The existence of these appeared to vary considerably.

  Some services told us they had written policies and guidelines in place. These covered issues such as obtaining informed consent, taking case histories, checking for possible contra-indications, and seeking permission of clinicians. Other services appeared not to have such policies or at least did not tell us of any.

- **Good literature and educational materials are available**

  Many providers appeared to have a good selection of resources, such as books and videos, available to patients. We have listed some of these in Appendix 2.

● **Therapies are offered to carers and staff too**

We were encouraged to see that many services offer therapies to staff and carers as well as patients. Caring for people with cancer can be physically and emotionally draining, and this inclusive approach to service provision is very welcome.

We hope to analyse further the patterns and trends that have emerged from the data.

Dr Michelle Kohn MB BSc MRCP

Project Chair and Complementary
Therapies Medical Adviser

Macmillan Cancer Relief
April 2002

References:

1. The *2001 Directory of Hospice and Palliative Care Services in the United Kingdom and Republic of Ireland* (2001). St Christopher's Hospice Information Service

2. *Directory of Cancer Self Help and Support* (2001/2), Cancerlink

3. *Cancer Care 2000: Comprehensive Review of Diagnostic & Screening Services, Treatment Centres and Palliative Care Services within the United Kingdom.* Cambridge Healthcare Publishing Ltd for Cambridge Cancer Research Fund

Complementary therapies – what you need to consider

Below is a checklist of practical steps that Macmillan recommends patients take to reassure themselves, before trying out a particular therapy or therapist. These draw on guidance issued by several cancer organisations.

DO ...

- Establish what the therapy is intended to achieve

- Use a therapist who has a recognised qualification, belongs to a professional body and has insurance. Ask if the person is experienced and/or trained in treating cancer patients

- Ask for an informal chat with the therapist, and/or ask for any leaflets or literature supplied by them

- Find out what the fees are (if any) and what these cover

- Talk to family, friends and health professionals

DON'T ...

- Abandon proven conventional treatments

- Be misled by promises or suggestions of cures or respond to a 'hard sell' that offers simple solutions

- Rely on a single source of information as it may be inaccurate

- Use a therapist who cannot refer you to the relevant research

- Feel pressured to buy expensive books, videos, nutritional supplements or herbal preparations as part of a therapy

- Be afraid to ask for references and credentials

- Consult any relevant fact sheets/telephone helplines provided by reputable patient support organisations

- Find out what is available on the NHS: in treatment centres you may already be using or through your family doctor at the Medical Centre. Wherever you are, ask about the availability of the full range of complementary therapy services

Personal recommendations are worth having, but should be considered only in addition to the above questions, not instead of them.

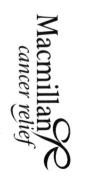

Macmillan
cancer relief

Registered Office 89 Albert Embankment, London SE1 7UQ
Tel: 020 7840 7840 Fax: 020 7840 7841 **Macmillan CancerLine 0808 808 2020**
www.macmillan.org.uk

Registered Charity Number 261017

Your comments

Dear Reader

We would really value your views and comments on how helpful you have found this directory and any changes or recommendations you would like to see incorporated into any further editions.

Please complete and return this form to us, either by post or email, at the address below:

Services Administration
Macmillan Cancer Relief, 89 Albert Embankment, London SE1 7UQ
Email: ctdirectory@macmillan.org.uk

Your name _____

Contact details _____

_____

Have you found the directory useful? (please give details)

_____

_____

_____

Is the directory easy to use?   Yes   No   (please circle)

Please specify what you liked/disliked about the directory?

_____

_____

How do you feel the directory could be improved?

_____

_____

If you have any questions regarding this directory please contact Services Administration
on 020 7840 4684

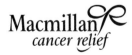

Registered Office 89 Albert Embankment, London SE1 7UQ
Tel: 020 7840 7840 Fax: 020 7840 7841 **Macmillan CancerLine 0808 808 2020**
www.macmillan.org.uk   *Registered Charity Number 261017*